Renal Diet Cookbook for Beginners

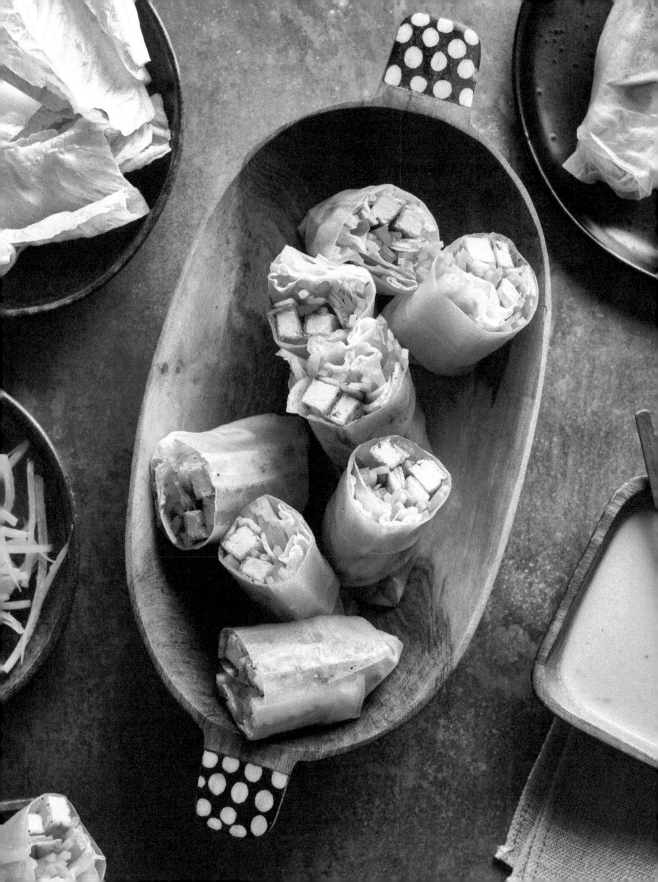

Renal Diet Cookbook
for Beginners

75 Simple Recipes to Help
Manage Chronic Kidney Disease

Edith Yang, RD, CSR, CLT

PHOTOGRAPHY BY DARREN MUIR

ROCKRIDGE
PRESS

Interior and Cover Designer: Stephanie Mautone
Art Producer: Meg Baggott
Editor: Rachelle Cihonski
Production Editor: Jenna Dutton
Production Manager: Jose Olivera

Photography ©2021 Darren Muir. Food styling by Yolanda Muir.

ISBN: Print 978-1-64876-632-9
eBook 978-1-64876-136-2
R0

To my husband, Tenny, and my parents,
Cindy and Steve, for inspiring, encouraging,
and supporting me in all my endeavors.

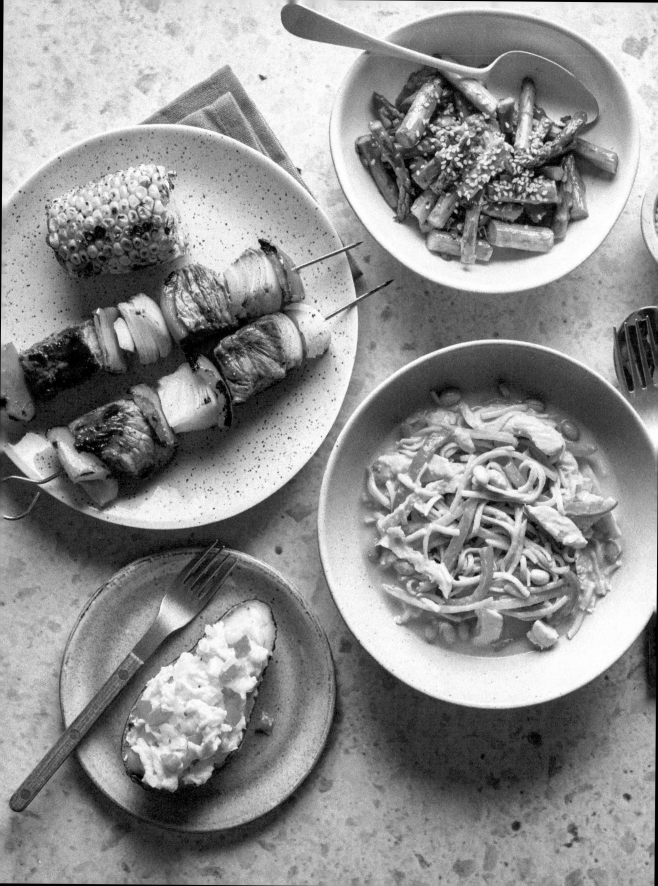

Contents

Introduction

Welcome to *Renal Diet Cookbook for Beginners*! My name is Edith Yang; I'm a registered dietitian who is board certified in renal nutrition. Chronic kidney disease (CKD) affects millions of people around the globe and most don't even know it. By picking up and reading this book, you are one step ahead of the game. My specialty is working with those who have CKD and helping them slow the progression of their kidney disease by making simple dietary and lifestyle changes. Though CKD may be scary and send you down a never-ending spiral of confusion and worry, you should rest assured knowing that CKD is a manageable health condition. My motto is "Healthy alternatives, infinite possibilities!" There is no one-size-fits-all approach to nutrition—my goal is to educate you on a kidney-friendly diet and provide you with the basic tools you need to make conscious and educated choices, and create a palatable, delicious, and nutritious diet to fit your lifestyle, needs, and tastes.

I've had many clients come to me at various stages of CKD, feeling very confused by all the information on the internet. Most of my clients don't even understand what is going on or why this is happening to them, and tell me that they are afraid to eat or are avoiding many foods. All of them are afraid of dialysis and want to avoid it. I've had much success providing medical nutrition therapy to help my clients delay the progression of the disease and improve their quality of life. Many of my clients have seen improvements in their kidney function with proper nutrition and lifestyle changes. Their success inspired me to write this book, so I could help those affected by CKD and their caregivers navigate through the confusing and conflicting information about the disease.

I believe that knowledge is power and that everyone should have access to and make informed choices about their health and wellness. There is a lot of outdated misinformation on the internet regarding the renal diet. This book will help clear up that information, help you understand the condition, and provide you with up-to-date and evidenced-based nutrition information. We will go through what CKD is, how it happens, and how you can manage it so that you can continue to live a fulfilling life and slow its progression.

The renal diet doesn't have to be boring and unpalatable. There are a plethora of recipes in this book that the whole family can enjoy. Most of the recipes are designed so that even the most beginner chefs can prepare them. The recipes have tips so that you can customize them to your specific tastes or preferences, and are modified to fit those with other comorbidities such as diabetes and hypertension.

The first step to taking control is educating yourself and you are doing just that!

Please note: *This book is written for those with CKD not yet on dialysis. The nutritional needs for those on dialysis are different. Furthermore, every person is different, and everyone has different nutrients they will need to monitor with CKD. You may be at the same stage of CKD as someone but have completely different dietary needs depending on your body and your overall condition. Your nutrition needs may also change as your CKD progresses or changes. The general guidelines in this book are not intended to treat, diagnose, or give specific medical advice. All of the content in this book was created by a board-certified registered dietitian and strives to provide only accurate, scientific-based information. However, your specific health needs may or may not apply. It is best to speak with your medical provider and/or registered dietitian regarding your specific nutrient needs or before starting any dietary protocol.*

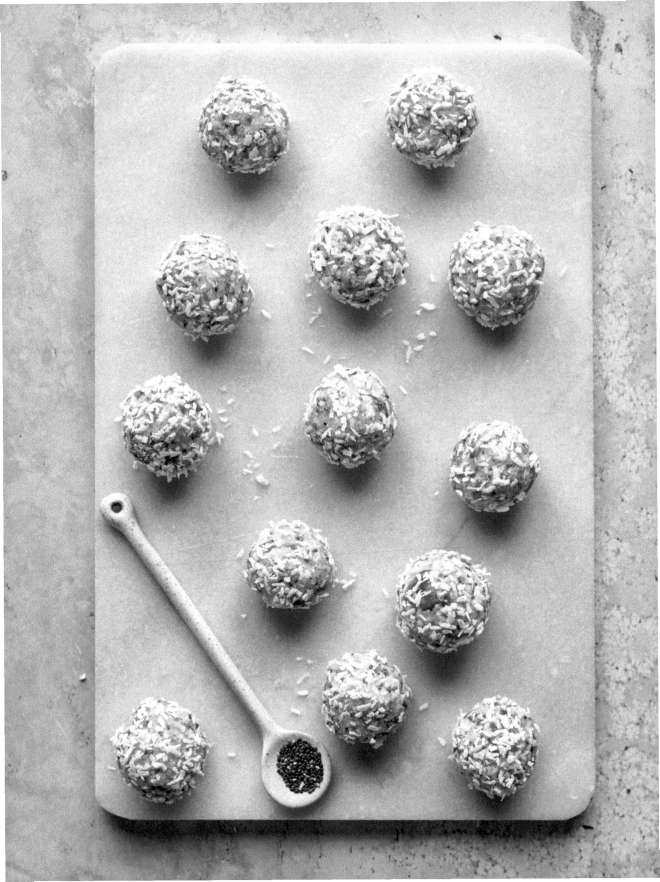

1
Understanding the Renal Diet

D iet and nutrition are crucial components of living with chronic kidney disease. What and how much we eat plays a large role in helping manage CKD. Following a kidney-friendly diet is extremely important and can help slow the advancement of your kidney disease. Depending on how well your kidneys are working or what stage of CKD you are in will determine what nutrients you will need to watch out for. It may seem complex and daunting, but this book will be your guide to help you manage CKD.

◁ Tangy Lemon Energy Bites, page 123

What Is Chronic Kidney Disease?

In 2019, it was estimated that more than 37 million adults in the United States have chronic kidney disease (CKD). Most people are unaware they have kidney disease until it progresses to the later stages and they start to show symptoms. But before we get into what CKD is and how it develops, let me first explain what the kidneys are and what they do.

The kidneys are bean-shaped, fist-size organs located symmetrically on either side of the spine. Each kidney weighs 4 to 6 ounces and contains more than half a million nephrons (filtering units). The kidneys have many important jobs, such as removing extra fluids and waste products, maintaining electrolyte balance, controlling blood pressure, helping make red blood cells, and keeping our bones healthy. Our kidneys work 24 hours a day to keep our bodies healthy and in balance. CKD occurs when the nephrons are damaged and can no longer do their job. As a result, toxins and fluids build up and cause more damage to the body.

The Causes of CKD

Diabetes and hypertension are the most common causes of CKD. Other factors that put people at risk for CKD are heart disease, family history of kidney disease, obesity, autoimmune diseases, overuse of painkillers, genetic disorders, kidney stones, and urinary tract infections. It's important to note that as we age, there is a normal decrease in our kidney function. After 30 years of age, our kidney function declines about 10 percent with each passing decade. This makes it even more important to monitor your kidney function and do what you can to slow its progression.

DIABETES

Diabetes is the number one cause of CKD in the US. If you have CKD caused by diabetes, it is commonly referred to as diabetic kidney disease (DKD) or diabetic nephropathy. Diabetes leads to CKD in various ways but generally it is due to high blood sugar. If your blood sugar is not under control and you have consistently high blood sugar levels, damage to the blood vessels in the nephrons of the kidneys occurs.

If you have diabetes, take control of your blood sugar and speak with your healthcare practitioner (HCP) and dietitian about what goals are best for you.

HYPERTENSION/HIGH BLOOD PRESSURE

The second leading cause of CKD is hypertension (HTN) or high blood pressure; these cases account for about 30 percent of all cases of end-stage kidney disease in the United States. HTN occurs when the pressure of blood against the walls of your blood vessels gets too high. Over time, high blood pressure damages your blood vessels and reduces blood flow to your organs, including the kidneys. HTN damages your nephrons and they become unable to properly filter out extra waste, toxins, and fluids.

Normal adult blood pressure is less than 120/80. Blood pressure goals for those with CKD should be as close to normal as possible. However, every person is different, so be sure to ask your HCP what goals are appropriate for you.

CARING FOR SOMEONE WITH CKD

Caring for someone with CKD can be a very complex, challenging, and stressful task. However, being a caregiver for someone with CKD is especially important, because many who are going through this are lost and overwhelmed. Having a good support system is crucial for the success and management of the disease.

The information and recipes in this book are designed to fit the needs of the person with CKD but they are also designed to fit the palates of everyone, including you. You may need to modify the way you currently cook and prepare foods, but know that the recipes are designed to be nutritious and benefit everyone while still being delicious. As caregivers and family members, you should keep an open mind and know that you can modify and adjust the taste profiles of the recipes after cooking by adding your own seasonings, spices, and sauces.

Living with kidney disease or caring for someone with it requires patience, courage, and positivity. Thank you for being a part of someone's life and helping them work through this disease.

Diagnosing CKD

As I mentioned earlier, most people don't realize they have kidney disease until it's very advanced. At the later stages of CKD, you may start to show symptoms such as water retention (edema), fatigue, itching, decreased appetite, sleep disturbances, anemia, and an increased sensitivity to medications. The best way to find out if you do have kidney disease is to have your healthcare practitioner run simple blood and urine tests. I recommend all adults with or without CKD to check in with their HCP at least once a year for a routine physical and to get blood work done.

In general, your HCP will want to evaluate your estimated glomerular filtration rate (eGFR), creatinine, and urine to assess and stage your CKD. The eGFR estimates how well your kidney's nephrons are filtering. You can think of the eGFR in terms of a percentage. If your eGFR is 87, your kidneys are working at 87 percent of their capacity. Most healthy adults have an eGFR of 90 mL/min/1.73m^2 or higher. The National Kidney Foundation defines CKD as having kidney damage or a decreased GFR for more than three months.

The First Steps

When you first find out you have CKD, your primary doctor or other HCP may talk to you about what caused your kidney disease. They will likely refer you to a nephrologist, but if not, you should ask for a referral. A nephrologist is a doctor who specializes in treating kidney disease, and can provide you with more detailed information on what you need to do to and guide you on the proper steps to help manage your condition.

Another specialist you should be referred to or request to see is a registered dietitian. A registered dietitian (RD/RDN) is someone who is trained in food and nutrition and how these things impact the body. They are able to provide you with medical nutrition therapy, which is important if you have CKD. A nutritionist or health coach is not the same thing as a dietitian. RD/RDNs must have a bachelors degree, take courses from an accredited program, undergo extensive training and complete more than 900 hours of supervised practice through an internship. In addition, they must take and pass a national exam that is overseen by the Commission on Dietetic Registration.

There are some registered dietitians, such as myself, who specialize in kidney nutrition. They are referred to as a CSR (board certified specialist in renal nutrition). You can refer to the Resources (page 148) to find a CKD dietitian near you. As you will learn throughout this book, diet and nutrition are critical in helping you manage your kidney disease. When you meet with a dietitian, they will go over your complete medical history, review your labs, medications, and any other pertinent health or lifestyle information and develop a plan personalized just for you. Though this book will provide a basic guideline for you, it is important to know that individual needs can vary and seeking out professional help is recommended.

The Five Stages

CKD is typically a progressive disease. Your kidney function declines over time. Knowing what stage you are in is one of the first steps toward managing the disease. There are five different stages of CKD and your diet and nutrition needs may vary at each stage.

STAGE	GFR (ML/MIN/1.73M²)	DESCRIPTION
1	$\geq$90	Near normal to mild kidney damage
2	60–89	Mild kidney damage
3a	45–59	Mild to moderate kidney damage
3b	30–44	Moderate to severe kidney damage
4	15–29	Severe kidney damage
5	<15	Kidney Failure

Stage 1 (GFR $\geq$90 mL/min/1.73m²)

This stage is typically considered normal kidney function. At this point, you want to make sure that your blood sugar and blood pressure are well controlled. You will want to work on your diet and make adjustments in your lifestyle as needed, such as quit smoking, maintain a healthy weight, and exercise regularly.

Stage 2 (GFR 60–89 mL/min/1.73m^2)

There is mild kidney damage, but your kidneys are still relatively healthy and able to do their job fairly well. You most likely won't even know you are at this stage as most don't show any symptoms yet. Your healthcare practitioner may want to check your urine and monitor your GFR periodically to see how the kidney disease is progressing. At this stage, make sure that your diet is nourishing and well-balanced, and that you quit smoking, exercise regularly, take your medications as prescribed, and have regular checkups with your doctor. If you have diabetes or hypertension, keep your blood sugar and blood pressure well controlled.

Stage 3a (GFR 45–59 mL/min/1.73m^2)

At this stage, you have mild to moderate kidney damage. Most people at this stage still don't show any signs or symptoms. Although if you do, you may experience fluid retention (edema) and changes in your urine. Making healthy lifestyle changes such as eating a well-balanced nutritious diet, habitually exercising, and maintaining a healthy weight are important components to help manage the disease. If you are diabetic or have hypertension, be sure to maintain your blood sugar and blood pressure in the appropriate ranges.

Stage 3b (GFR 30–44 mL/min/1.73m^2)

Your kidney disease has progressed, and the damage is moderate to severe. You should be working with a nephrologist to develop a more specialized treatment plan. At this point in the disease, you want to make sure you are eating a diet with appropriate protein content, limiting sodium intake, and cutting back on excess sugars and saturated fats. Also, if you haven't already, you should be keeping your blood sugar and blood pressure under control, quit smoking, and maintain a healthy lifestyle that includes regular exercise of at least 150 minutes per week.

At stages 3a and 3b, you should definitely talk to your doctor about seeing a dietitian or search for one on your own. Diet and proper nutrition are a crucial part of delaying the progression of your kidney disease.

Stage 4 (GFR 15–29 mL/min/1.73m²)

At this stage, your kidneys are severely damaged and working at less than 30 percent capacity. You are most likely showing symptoms of CKD such as fluid retention, tiredness, foamy urine, back pain, nausea and vomiting, changes in taste, and loss of appetite. Though the disease is at a later stage, you can still work at your diet and lifestyle to slow its progression. If you aren't already seeing a nephrologist, you definitely want to ask your primary healthcare provider to refer you to one. During this stage, you and your doctor may want to discuss treatment options and you should be working with a dietitian if you aren't already. Diet and maintaining a healthy lifestyle are critical at this point to slow down the progression of your CKD. Be sure you are communicating with your doctor, taking your medications as prescribed, and are always prepared for your appointments. At this stage, your doctor is likely monitoring your labs and urine more frequently. Be proactive, participate in your care, and ask questions if needed.

Stage 5 (GFR <15 mL/min/1.73m²)

This stage is known as end-stage or kidney failure. Your kidneys are working at less than 15 percent of their capacity, meaning that they have lost nearly all their functional abilities. If you haven't already been experiencing symptoms, you most likely are having them at this stage. Common symptoms that occur at this point are loss of appetite, changes in weight due to fluid retention, fatigue, headaches or difficulty concentrating, itching, decreased urine output, and tingling in your hands and feet. Toxins are building up in your body and causing you to feel ill.

Once your nephrons are damaged, they usually don't recover completely, but don't panic. Although there is no cure for kidney disease, there are definitely things you can do to take control of the disease and delay its progression. You can still live a happy and quality life by making appropriate changes in your diet and lifestyle.

What to Expect on the Renal Diet

Every person is different, and everyone has different nutrients they will need to monitor with CKD. You may be at the same stage of CKD as someone but have completely different diet needs depending on your body and your overall condition.

The CKD diet requires you, your healthcare practitioner, and hopefully also a dietitian to monitor your labs and progress to ensure you are following an appropriate diet. While it may be overwhelming to think about all the different components, the diet is manageable if you have the proper tools and guidance. The fact that you are reading this book is a great sign that you are on the right path. You may feel overwhelmed or think that this diet is going to be terrible, but I promise you there are plenty of tasty recipes that can be created on a renal diet.

The renal diet includes a variety of whole grains, appropriate proteins, plenty of fruits and vegetables, and flavorful and fun seasoning and spices. There are certain nutrients that people with CKD may need to watch out for; these may include, but are not limited to, protein, potassium, phosphorus, and sodium. While these nutrients are important to monitor depending on your needs, it's also good to note that there are many foods you can incorporate into your diet that are tasty as well as nutritious and good for your body.

Protein

Protein is considered the building block of life. It is part of our muscle, skin, hair, and nails. Our bodies need protein to grow and develop, help repair tissues, fight infections, and heal from injuries. Though protein is important, those with CKD need to be mindful of protein intake. When we eat protein, our body metabolizes it and uses it but some of it also becomes waste products. Healthy kidneys are able to filter these waste products and excrete them in our urine. However, those with CKD are not able to remove the wastes as effectively, and the waste ends up building up in our blood. When you have too much protein in your body, it puts extra stress onto the kidneys and makes it even harder to remove the waste products. When you have CKD, your protein needs will be different and likely less than usual.

There are two different types of protein—animal proteins and plant proteins. Animal proteins (beef, chicken, fish, pork, dairy, eggs) are considered high-biological value because they contain a sufficient number of amino acids, which are the components of protein that our body needs. Though they are considered high-quality proteins, animal proteins create more waste products in our bodies than plant proteins and our kidneys are not able to filter them as well. Plant proteins don't create as much waste product when our body metabolizes them and therefore put less strain on our kidneys. Newer research is showing that following a more plant-based diet has been beneficial for those with CKD. Examples of plant proteins are nuts, nut butters, seeds, tofu, grains, beans, lentils, peas, soy, and tempeh.

PROTEIN CONTENT IN COMMON FOODS

EGGS, MEAT, POULTRY, SEAFOOD*	NUTS AND SEEDS**	LEGUMES AND VEGETABLES***	CEREAL, BREADS, AND GRAINS	DAIRY, SOY, NON-DAIRY MILK BEVERAGES
· Beef · Chicken · Clams · Egg (1 large) · Fish · Lamb · Lobster (1.5 oz) · Pork · Salmon · Scallops (1.5 oz) · Shrimp · Tuna · Turkey	· Almonds · Brazil nuts (4g) · Cashews (5g) · Chia seeds (5g) · Flaxseed · Hazelnuts (4g) · Macadamia nuts (2g) · Peanuts (7g) · Peanut butter (1 tbsp = 7g) · Pecans (3g) · Pistachios · Pumpkin seeds (9g) · Soy nuts (12g) · Sunflower seeds · Walnuts (4g)	· Adzuki beans (9g) · Asparagus (2g) · Black beans (8g) · Black-eyed peas (7g) · Brussels sprouts (2g) · Chickpeas (7g) · Edamame (9g) · Fava beans (7g) · Green peas (4g) · Lentils (9g) · Lima beans (6g) · Pinto beans (11g) · Red kidney beans (8g) · Spinach (3g)	· Bagel (1 whole = 10g) · Biscuit (1 whole = 4g) · Brown rice (1 cup = 5g) · Corn tortilla (1g) · Flour tortilla (4g) · Hamburger bun (1 bun = 4g) · Macaroni (2 cups = 7g) · Pancakes (1 (6-inch) = 5g) · Popcorn (1 oz = 3g) · Quinoa (4g) · Spaghetti noodles (1 cup = 8g) · Waffles (1 (7-inch) = 6g) · White bread (1 slice = 3g) · White rice (1 cup = 4g) · Whole-wheat bread (1 slice = 4g)	· Almond milk (1 cup = 1g) · Cheese (blue cheese, Cheddar, Gouda, Gruyère, mozzarella, Colby, Swiss) (1 oz = about 7g) · Cottage cheese (1 oz = 4g) · Feta cheese (1 oz = 4g) · Greek yogurt (6 oz = 18g) · Milk (whole, low-fat, nonfat) (1 cup = 8g) · Oat milk (1 cup = 4g) · Parmesan cheese (1 oz = 11g) · Regular yogurt (1 cup = 11g) · Rice milk (1 cup = 1g) · Soy milk (1 cup = 7g) · String cheese (1 piece = 6g)

*One serving = 1 ounce and provides about 7 grams of protein unless otherwise indicated.
**One serving = 1 ounce and provides about 6 grams of protein unless otherwise indicated.
***One serving = ½ cup cooked unless otherwise indicated. Protein content varies.

Sodium

Sodium is an essential part of our lives and is needed by our bodies to function properly. Sodium helps us regulate blood pressure and maintain fluid balance. Although we need sodium, too much of it is harmful to the kidneys. If you have CKD, your kidneys can't get rid of the extra sodium or fluid. When these things build up, your blood pressure increases, and you may experience swelling and have difficulty breathing. Too much sodium and fluids in your body can also damage other organs.

Sodium is in almost everything you eat. You need to be especially careful about the amount of sodium you have in your diet. The recommended guidelines for sodium are less than 2,300 mg per day, which is equal to about 1 teaspoon of salt per day.

Avoid eating out whenever possible, since restaurant foods tend to be higher in sodium. Sometimes, something might not taste salty, but it can still be very high in sodium. If you do dine out, ask for sauces and dressings on the side and request no added salt on your food. Check food labels and the serving sizes to make sure you are sticking to your sodium goals. As a general guide, find foods that have 5 percent or less DV of sodium or <140 mg of sodium.

SODIUM CONTENT IN COMMON FOODS

	AVOID/LIMIT	CHOOSE
Vegetables	Canned or frozen vegetables that are seasoned or sauced, pickled or fermented vegetables	Fresh or frozen vegetables that are not pre-seasoned or pre-sauced, unsalted or low-sodium canned vegetables
Fruit	Canned in syrup	Fresh or frozen

SODIUM CONTENT IN COMMON FOODS

	AVOID/LIMIT	CHOOSE
Breads, Cereals, Starches	Instant hot cereals, quick breads, premade pan-cake/waffle/bread mixes, salted crackers/chips Rice, pasta, grain box mixes that are pre-seasoned or come with a seasoning packet Instant noodles	Make your own breads at home or buy from the bakery section—choose items that have a lower sodium content Plain rice, pasta, noodles, grains
Dairy	Processed cheeses, cheese spreads, butter-milk, instant pudding mix	Low-sodium cheese, milk, yogurt
Meat, Fish, Poultry	Cured meats, deli lunch meats, canned meats, bacon, sausages, corned beef, hot dogs, Spam	Fresh meat, fish, poultry, low- or no-sodium deli meats (can usually be found at the deli counter)
Snack Foods	Salted chips, crackers, popcorn, pretzels, pumpkin or sunflower seeds	Unsalted chips, crackers, popcorn, pretzels, seeds
Herbs and Seasonings	Salts (table/kosher/sea/Himalayan/flavored), MSG	No-salt seasonings (Mrs. Dash, Chef Paul Prudhomme) lemon, basil, oregano, parsley, turmeric, onion powder, garlic powder, cayenne pepper, black pepper, etc.
Sauces and Marinades	Salad dressings, barbe-cue sauce, ketchup, soy sauce, steak sauce, teriyaki sauce	No-salt-added sauces, marinades, and salad dressings (try making your own at home), lemon juice, mustard, Siete hot sauce, vinegar
Canned and Frozen Packaged Foods	Avoid all types of regular canned foods and frozen packaged meals	Low or no-salt-added canned goods; make big batches of recipes at home and freeze in appropriate portions for your own frozen meals

Potassium

Potassium is a mineral that helps keep our heartbeat regular and our muscles contracting properly. The kidneys play a role in making sure that we have the right amount of potassium in our bodies. With CKD, you may not be able to maintain proper potassium balance. Having too much or too little potassium can cause serious heart complications. Potassium is measured by a blood test; a normal blood potassium level is between 3.5 and 5.0 mEq/L. Though you may have CKD, you may or may not need to restrict your potassium intake. Your healthcare practitioner will review your labs to determine your potassium needs. Do not restrict unnecessarily, because there are complications that can occur if you don't have enough potassium in your diet. Foods that are high in potassium are also high in fiber, vitamins, minerals, and other nutrients we need. Potassium is mostly found in fruits, vegetables, legumes, nuts, meats, and dairy products. You may even find potassium in some salt substitutes, so be careful if you need to limit your intake.

POTASSIUM CONTENT IN COMMON FOODS*

LOW POTASSIUM (<200 mg/serving)			HIGH POTASSIUM (>200 mg/serving)		
Fruits	**Vegetables**	**Other Foods**	**Fruits**	**Vegetables**	**Other Foods**
· Apple (1 medium) · Applesauce · Blackberries · Blueberries · Cherries · Cranberries · Grapes · Grapefruit · Lemon/lime · Mandarin oranges	· Alfalfa sprouts · Asparagus (6 raw medium spears) · Beans, green or wax · Broccoli · Cabbage · Carrots · Cauliflower · Celery	· Cookies without nuts or chocolate · Noodles · Pasta · Pies without chocolate or high-potassium fruits · Rice	· Apricot, raw (2 medium), dried (5 halves) · Avocado (½ whole) · Banana (½ whole) · Cantaloupe · Coconut (1 cup) · Dates (5 whole) · Dried fruits	· Acorn squash · Artichoke · Baked beans · Bamboo shoots · Beet greens · Beets · Black beans · Broccoli, cooked · Bok choy	· Bran/bran products · Chocolate (2 ounces) · Granola · Milk (1 cup) · Molasses (1 tablespoon) · Nuts and seeds · Peanut butter (2 tablespoons) · Salt substitutes · Yogurt

*Serving size is ½ cup unless otherwise indicated.

POTASSIUM CONTENT IN COMMON FOODS*

LOW POTASSIUM (<200 mg/serving)			HIGH POTASSIUM (>200 mg/serving)		
Fruits	**Vegetables**	**Other Foods**	**Fruits**	**Vegetables**	**Other Foods**
· Peaches, fresh (1 small), canned (½ cup)	· Corn (½ ear fresh, ½ cup frozen)		· Grapefruit juice	· Brussels sprouts	
· Pears, fresh (1 small); canned (½ cup)	· Cucumber		· Honeydew	· Butternut squash	
· Pineapple	· Eggplant		· Kiwi (1 medium)	· Chinese cabbage	
· Plums (1 whole)	· Green peas		· Mango (1 medium)	· Dried beans	
· Raspberries	· Kale		· Orange (1 medium)	· French fries	
· Strawber-ries	· Lettuce		· Orange juice	· Kohlrabi	
· Tangerine (1 whole)	· Leeks		· Papaya (½ whole)	· Legumes	
· Watermelon (limit to 1 cup max)	· Mustard		· Pomegran-ate (1 whole)	· Lentils	
	· Parsley		· Pomegran-ate juice	· Lima beans	
	· Peppers		· Prunes	· Mushrooms, cooked	
	· Radish		· Prune juice	· Okra	
	· Rhubarb			· Parsnip	
	· Scallions			· Potatoes	
	· Spaghetti squash			· Pumpkin	
	· Spinach, raw			· Refried beans	
	· Water chestnuts, canned			· Spinach, cooked	
	· Yellow squash			· Swiss chard	
	· Zucchini			· Tomatoes	
				· Turnips	
				· Vegetable juices	

*Serving size is ½ cup unless otherwise indicated.

Phosphorus

Phosphorus is another essential mineral that the body needs. Most of the phosphorus in our bodies is found in the bones. Phosphorus helps us build strong bones and teeth, create energy, and produce hormones.

In the later stages of CKD, you may need to limit your phosphorus intake since the kidneys are not able to filter excess amounts out. Too much phosphorus can lead to bone disease and increase your risk of cardiovascular events. However, just like all the other nutrients, everyone's needs are different. You will want to closely monitor your labs and work with your dietitian and nephrologist to find out what your specific needs may be. A normal blood phosphorus level is between 2.7 and 4.6 mg/dl.

Phosphorus is found in almost all foods. We tend to absorb less phosphorus from plant-based than animal-based foods. Phosphorus used as a food additive is almost 100 percent absorbed by our bodies. Phosphate additives are commonly used in fast foods, ready-to-eat convenience foods, sodas, beverages, and enhanced meats—all of which are highly processed foods.

If your phosphorus levels are elevated, your doctor may prescribe a phosphorus binder that you need to take with meals to help you get rid of excess phosphorus.

PHOSPHORUS CONTENT IN COMMON FOODS*

LOW PHOSPHORUS (< 150 mg/serving)	MEDIUM PHOSPHORUS (151–250 mg/serving)	HIGH PHOSPHORUS (> 251 mg/serving)
· Apple	· Beans, black, 1 cup	· Almonds, oil/dry roasted, 2 ounces
· Bagel, 1 plain (4-inch diameter)	· Beans, fava, 1 cup	· Baked beans, 1 cup
· Barley, pearled, cooked	· Beans, kidney, 1 cup	· Beans, small white, mature, boiled, 1 cup
· Beans, green	· Beans, pinto, 1 cup	· Beef, liver, cooked, 3 ounces
· Bread, pita, 1 (6.5-inch diameter)	· Beef, bottom round, 3 ounces	· Beefalo, 3 ounces
· Bread, pumpernickel, 2 slices	· Beef, chuck roast, 3 ounces	· Buttermilk, 1 cup
· Bread, white, 2 slices	· Beef, eye round, 3 ounces	· Calamari, fried, 3 ounces
· Butter, 1 tablespoon	· Beef, ground, 70% lean, 3 ounces	
	· Beef, ground, 95% lean, 3 ounces	

*One serving = ½ cup unless otherwise indicated.

PHOSPHORUS CONTENT IN COMMON FOODS*

LOW PHOSPHORUS (< 150 mg/serving)	MEDIUM PHOSPHORUS (151–250 mg/serving)	HIGH PHOSPHORUS (> 251 mg/serving)
· Cabbage · Cauliflower · Cereal, crispy rice, 1 cup · Cheese, Brie, 1 ounce · Cheese, feta, 1 ounce · Cocoa, unsweetened, 2 tablespoons · Cookies, shortbread, 4 · Cornflakes, 1 cup · Cottage cheese, nonfat · Couscous, cooked · Cream cheese, 1 ounce · Cucumber · Duck, with skin, 3 ounces · Egg white, 1 large · Egg yolk, 1 large · Eggplant · English muffin, 1 plain · Figs · Gelatin, water base · Ginger ale, 1 can · Grapefruit · Grapes · Grouper · Hominy grits · Ice cream, 10% fat, vanilla · Lettuce · Milk, soy, 1 cup · Oatmeal, cooked, 1 packet · Onions · Oysters, canned, 3 ounces · Oysters, raw, Pacific, 3 ounces	· Beef, sirloin steak, 3 ounces · Black-eyed peas, 1 cup · Bread, whole-wheat, 2 slices · Catfish, breaded/fried, 3 ounces · Cheese, blue, 2 ounces · Cheese, Cheddar, 1 ounce · Cheese, mozzarella, 1 ounce · Cheese, provolone, 2 ounces · Cheese, Swiss, 1 ounce · Chicken, breast, 3 ounces · Chicken, dark meat, 3 ounces · Chickpeas, 1 cup · Chocolate, plain, 2 ounces · Cod, Pacific, 3 ounces · Cottage cheese, 1% fat · Cottage cheese, 2% fat · Crab, blue, cooked with moist heat, 3 ounces · Crab, Dungeness, cooked with moist heat, 3 ounces · Lamb, kebabs, domestic, 3 ounces · Lamb, leg roast, domestic, 3 ounces · Lamb, New Zealand, 3 ounces · Lobster, cooked with moist heat, 3 ounces · Macadamia nuts, 3 ounces	· Cashews, dry roasted, 2 ounces · Cereal, bran, 100% · Cereal, wheat-germ, ¼ cup · Cheese, goat, 2 ounces · Cheese, Parmesan, 2 ounces · Cheese, ricotta, part skim · Cheese, Romano, 2 ounces · Chia seeds, 1 ounce · Chicken, liver, cooked, 3 ounces · Clam chowder, New England · Clams, cooked with moist heat, 3 ounces · Corn bread, 1 piece · Crab, Alaska king, cooked with moist heat, 3 ounces · Custard, flan, 1 cup · Flounder, 3 ounces · Halibut, Atlantic/Pacific, 3 ounces · Lentils, mature, boiled, 1 cup · Milk, 1%, 1 cup · Milk, chocolate, 1 cup · Milk, evaporated, nonfat · Milk, nonfat, 1 cup · Milk, whole, 1 cup · Mussels, blue, cooked with moist heat, 3 ounces · Nuts, Brazil, 2 ounces · Nuts, pine, 2 ounces

*One serving = ½ cup unless otherwise indicated.

CONTINUED ▶

PHOSPHORUS CONTENT IN COMMON FOODS*

LOW PHOSPHORUS (< 150 mg/serving)	MEDIUM PHOSPHORUS (151–250 mg/serving)	HIGH PHOSPHORUS (> 251 mg/serving)
· Pasta, 1 cup · Peas, split, mature, boiled · Plums · Popcorn, air-popped, 1 cup · Pork, spare ribs, 3 ounces · Radishes · Rice cakes, 1 cake · Rice, white, enriched, cooked · Sherbet · Shrimp, cooked with moist heat, 3 ounces · Sour cream · Tofu, soft · Wheat flour, white, 1 cup	· Milk, canned, sweetened, condensed, ¼ cup · Mushrooms, cooked, 1 cup · Mussels, raw, blue, 3 ounces · Peanut butter, 2 tablespoons · Pork, boneless loin chop, 3 ounces · Pork, leg roast, 3 ounces · Raisin Bran, 1 cup · Raisins, seedless, 1 cup · Rice, brown, cooked, 1 cup · Shredded Wheat, 1 cup · Shrimp, breaded/fried, 3 ounces · Snapper, 3 ounces · Spinach, raw · Tortilla, 2 corn or flour (6-inch diameter) · Turkey, breast, 3 ounces · Turkey, dark meat, 3 ounces · Veal, rib roast, 3 ounces · Wheat flakes, 1 cup	· Oysters, Eastern, cooked with moist heat, 3 ounces · Peanuts, boiled, 1 cup · Peanuts, dry roasted, 3 ounces · Peanuts, oil roasted, 2 ounces · Pecans, oil/dry roasted, 3 ounces · Salmon, canned, pink/red, 3 ounces · Sardines, canned in oil, 3 ounces · Scallops, breaded/fried, 3 ounces · Sole, 3 ounces · Soybeans, mature, boiled · Sunflower seeds, 1 ounce · Swordfish, 3 ounces · Tofu, raw, firm · Tuna, light, canned in oil, 3 ounces · Tuna, white, canned in oil, 3 ounces · Veal, cubed, stewed, 3 ounces · Walnuts, English, 2 ounces · Wheat flour, whole-grain, 1 cup · Yogurt, low-fat · Yogurt, skim

*One serving = ½ cup unless otherwise indicated.

Eat More of the Good Stuff

The kidney-friendly diet requires that you pay attention to certain nutrients to avoid overworking your kidneys and causing more damage to the body. While you may have to monitor or be more mindful of certain nutrients, there are other foods that you can and should incorporate more of into your diet.

Healthy Carbohydrates and Whole Grains

Carbohydrates provide your body with the energy it needs to function properly. Glucose, which is a carbohydrate, is the preferred source of fuel for our brains. There are different types of carbohydrates—starches, sugars, and fiber—and all types can be a part of a healthy diet.

When including carbohydrates in your diet, it is important to include whole grains. In the past, whole grains were not recommended for those with kidney disease because of their high phosphorus content. However, newer research has found that the phosphorus in whole grains is not broken down and absorbed as easily in the human body. Whole grains are those that have been harvested in their complete form and includes the endosperm, bran, and germ of the grain. Because whole grains are minimally processed, they provide a ton of nutrients, including fiber, vitamins, and minerals. Examples of whole grains include oats, barley, quinoa, popcorn, and brown rice. When choosing your carbohydrates, be sure to read the back of the package where the food ingredients are listed to find the words "whole wheat" or "whole grain." Be careful of the claims on the front of the package, because they can be misleading.

It is recommended that at least half of your carbohydrates come from whole-grain sources. If you are using the plate method to prepare your meals, a quarter of your plate should consist of healthy carbohydrates.

CARBOHYDRATES AND DIABETES

When you have diabetes, being consistent with your carbohydrate intake is very important. Many people think that having diabetes means that you have to cut out carbohydrates. However, this is far from the truth. As I mentioned, carbohydrates provide you with energy and they are essential for your body to work properly and efficiently. When you have diabetes, you still need carbohydrates to function. You will want to make sure to monitor how many carbohydrates you eat and be sure to include healthy whole grains in your diet. Remember that controlling your blood sugar is important when you have CKD. Work closely with your dietitian and doctor to figure out the specific amount of carbohydrates you should eat daily to meet your blood sugar goals.

Fruits and Vegetables

Fruits and vegetables are an important component of a renal diet. I'm sure your internet search so far on the renal diet has scared you into thinking you can't eat a lot of them due to the potassium content. Remember, potassium is generally not restricted for those with CKD unless indicated. Work closely with your nephrologist and renal dietitian to ensure that you are following the plan that is best for you. Fruits and vegetables have so many health benefits—they provide fiber, vitamins, and minerals. They can also help with weight management and lowering your blood pressure. Because of their numerous health benefits, fruits and vegetables don't put as much stress on your kidneys as other foods, such as animal proteins, so it's a good idea to include them in your diet. Try to fill half of your plate with fruits and vegetables—a colorful plate indicates a wide variety of nutrients.

If you do need to watch out for potassium, pay attention to the high/low potassium foods list (page 12) and make sure to keep track of your intake using the daily food log tracker (page 23).

HIGH-FIBER FOODS

Fiber is especially important for those with CKD, because as kidney function declines, your ability to get rid of toxins decreases. Fiber helps with your gut health, which in turn can help you get rid of some of the toxins that are building up in your body. Low fiber intake is correlated with increased inflammation and an elevated risk of heart disease. The standard American diet is generally low in fiber, which is not good for your overall health. The recommended daily fiber intake for women under 50 years old is >25 grams per day and older than 51 years old is >21 grams per day. Men under 50 years old need >38 grams of fiber per day and older than 51 years old need >28 grams per day.

Whole grains, fruits, and vegetables are examples of high-fiber foods, so be sure to include these good things in your diet. Some kidney-friendly options include jicama, eggplant, kale, chickpeas, berries, plums, chia seeds, flaxseed, and whole-grain cereals.

FIBER CONTENT IN COMMON FOODS*

FRUITS	VEGETABLES	GRAINS	PROTEINS
· Apple, 1 medium, 4g · Avocado, ½ medium, 4.5g · Banana, 1 medium, 3g · Blackberries, 4g · Blueberries, 2g · Cherries, 1.5g · Grapes, 7.5g · Jicama, 3g · Pear, 1 medium, 6g · Raspberries, 4g · Strawberries, 1.5g	· Broccoli, cooked, 2.5g · Brussels sprouts, cooked, 3g · Cauliflower, cooked, 2.5g · Collard greens, cooked, 2.5g · Kale, cooked, 1.5g · Mustard greens, cooked, 2.5g · Peas, frozen, 7g · Spinach, cooked, 2g · Spaghetti squash, 1.5g · Sweet potato, 1 medium, 4g · Swiss chard, cooked 2g · Zucchini, 1.5g	· Barley, pearled, cooked, 3g · Brown rice, cooked, 2g · Oats, dry, 4g · Popcorn, air-popped, 3 cups, 4g · Quinoa, cooked, 2.5g · Wasa crispbread, 2 slices, 4g · Whole-wheat bread, 1 slice, 2g · Whole-wheat pasta, cooked, 3g · Wild rice, cooked, 1.5g	· Almonds, 1 oz, 4g · Black beans, 7.5g · Broad beans, 4.5g · Chickpeas, 6g · Edamame, 3g · Kidney beans, 8g · Lentils, 8g · Mung beans, 7.5g · Navy beans, 9.5g · Peanuts, 1 oz, 2g · Pinto beans, 7.5g · Pumpkin seeds, 3g · Sunflower seeds, ¼ cup, 3g · Walnuts, 1 oz, 2g · White beans, 9.5g

*One serving = ½ cup, unless otherwise indicated.

Healthy Fats

Fat is another macronutrient that has a bad reputation. For many years, many people thought that eating fat makes you fat. However, this is not the case. Fat is a macronutrient that you need, and it should compose 20 to 35 percent of your daily calorie intake. Fat helps promote normal functioning of the brain and nervous system, maintain cholesterol levels, and reduce inflammation, all of which are important in CKD. When including fats in your diet, you want to limit your intake of "bad" fats (aka saturated and trans fats) and choose "good" fats (aka unsaturated fats).

Sources of saturated fats include hydrogenated oils, animal proteins, cheese, butter, and whole- or reduced-fat milk dairy products.

Sources of unsaturated fats include fatty fish such as salmon, walnuts, chia seeds, eggs, olive oil, avocadoes and avocado oil, and peanut butter.

It is recommended to use olive oil or avocado oil when cooking or making dressings, sauces, and marinades. Also, unsalted nut butters or a proper serving of nuts as a snack is a delicious way to get some healthy fats in your diet. Fat is calorie dense, so a little goes a long way.

Other Things to Keep in Mind

While diet is a crucial component of managing your kidney disease, there are other factors that you should also pay attention to for your overall health and wellness.

Medications: Be sure to let your nephrologist know about all the medications you are taking. There may be some medications that are not compatible with your kidneys depending on what stage of CKD you are at. You also want to make sure that you are taking all appropriate medications as prescribed by your doctor. Any time you have a change in medications by any healthcare practitioner, it is a good idea to let your nephrologist and dietitian know.

Vitamins and minerals: There are some vitamins and minerals that are not appropriate for those with CKD and may build up to a toxic level in your body. What vitamin and mineral supplements you can or cannot take depends on what stage you are at and how well your kidneys are functioning. Be sure to tell your nephrologist and dietitian about what supplements you are taking so that they can make adjustments as needed.

Quit smoking: It is no secret that smoking is dangerous to the human body. For many years, the US surgeon general and CDC have warned the public about the negative effects that smoking has on every part of the body, including the kidneys and the advancement of CKD. Smoking damages the cardiovascular system, causes increases in blood pressure and heart rate, and reduces blood flow to the kidneys. If you smoke, it's important to quit.

Exercise: It is recommended that adults partake in at least 150 minutes of moderate-intensity or 75 minutes of vigorous-intensity exercise per week. Everyone should engage in regular physical activity unless otherwise indicated by a doctor or other healthcare professional. Exercise is very important especially if you have CKD.

It can help you maintain a healthy weight, improve your blood pressure and blood sugar, build strength and endurance, and even aid your sleep. Choose exercise activities that you enjoy and are appropriate for your age, physical condition, and abilities.

Nutritional Needs by Stage

CKD nutritional needs usually vary based on a person's current stage of kidney disease. Everyone is different, however, and your healthcare practitioner may adjust your needs based on your current age, weight, labs, and overall health condition.

NUTRITIONAL NEEDS BY STAGE

CKD STAGE	PROTEIN	SODIUM	PHOSPHORUS	POTASSIUM
Stage 1–2	0.8–1.2 grams of protein per kilogram of ideal body weight (see chart page 22)	<2,300mg	Maintain a blood phosphorus level that is within the normal range	Maintain a blood potassium level that is within the normal range
Stage 3	0.55–0.6 grams of protein per kilogram of ideal body weight	<2,300mg	Maintain a blood phosphorus level that is within the normal range	Maintain a blood potassium level that is within the normal range
Stage 4	Protein needs may vary depending on your personal needs/goals—talk to your dietitian and nephrologist about what is right for you	Sodium needs may vary depending on your personal needs/goals—talk to your dietitian and nephrologist about what is right for you	Based on your labs, you may need to restrict phosphorus to 800–1000 mg/day	Based on your labs, you may need to adjust your potassium intake—talk to your dietitian and nephrologist about what is right for you
*Stage 5 (non-dialysis)				

*Stage 5 (non-dialysis): The nutrition needs at this stage are very specific and must be tailored to the unique individual. A thorough evaluation by your renal dietitian is recommended to create a personal plan of care.

For Diabetes: If you have diabetes and CKD, your protein needs can be slightly higher at 0.8 to 0.9 grams of protein per kilogram of body weight. Diabetics have an increased protein requirement to help with blood sugar control.

Example: For a 5-foot-2-inch-tall woman with stage 3 CKD, the estimated ideal body weight is 50 kilograms. You would estimate your daily protein needs by multiplying 0.55 grams of protein by 50 kilograms: *0.55 grams of protein x 50 kilograms = 27.5 grams of protein per day.*

IDEAL BODY WEIGHT

MALE		FEMALE	
HEIGHT	IBW (KG)	HEIGHT	IBW (KG)
5 ft	48	4 ft 10	41
5 ft 1	51	4 ft 11	43
5 ft 2	54	5 ft	45
5 ft 3	56	5 ft 1	48
5 ft 4	59	5 ft 2	50
5 ft 5	62	5 ft 3	52
5 ft 6	65	5 ft 4	55
5 ft 7	67	5 ft 5	57
5 ft 8	70	5 ft 6	59
5 ft 9	73	5 ft 7	61
5 ft 10	75	5 ft 8	64
5 ft 11	78	5 ft 9	66
6 ft	81	5 ft 10	68
6 ft 1	84	5 ft 11	70
6 ft 2	86	6 ft	73
6 ft 3	89		
6 ft 4	92		

The weights listed in this table provide a quick estimate of your lean body mass. Your ideal body weight may be higher or lower than the weight listed in this table. Many factors go into determining an individual's ideal body weight, and so you should consult your HCP for more specific guidance.

Personalizing Your Nutrition

As I've mentioned many times throughout this chapter, every person is unique and may have different nutrition requirements. Be proactive in your care and work closely with your nephrologist and renal dietitian to find out what your specific needs/goals should be to help you manage CKD. Use this chart to keep track of your needs and any special components you need to make note of.

NUTRIENT	MY NEEDS/GOALS	NOTES
Protein	*Example: 5-foot 2-inch woman with stage 3 CKD* *27.5 grams of protein per day*	*Limit animal proteins*
Sodium		
Potassium		
Phosphorus		
Carbohydrates		
Fats		
Vitamins/Minerals		
Blood Sugar		
Blood Pressure		

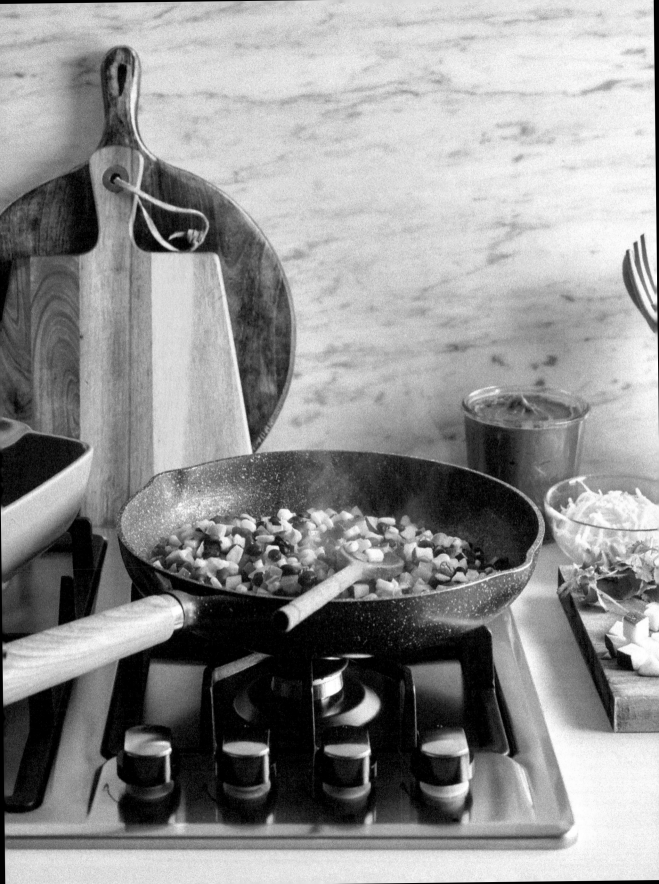

2

Cooking Basics

Cooking doesn't have to be difficult and once you learn the basics, you will find that cooking can be easy and fun. The recipes in this book are perfect for beginners and don't require any fancy equipment, extensive skills, or training. With a bit of planning and preparing, you can easily master a variety of different recipes and techniques.

Getting Started

The first step is to read the recipe entirely before you start cooking to prevent making any mistakes while cooking or baking. When reading, take note of what ingredients or equipment you might need. You will also want to take note of the preparation time and recipe yield (does it make enough, or do you need to double or halve it?). I find it helpful to read through a recipe twice: first to check if the recipe meets my needs, and second to prepare all my ingredients and arrange them in order to be more efficient when cooking starts.

The most important tips are to have fun and be confident. Cooking can be an enjoyable and therapeutic activity for you and your family. Don't be afraid of trying new things and experimenting with different tastes and flavors!

Essential Kitchen Tools

Before beginning any cooking adventure, you need to have the proper equipment so that you can seamlessly prepare your meals and snacks. Kitchen tools don't have to be fancy; you can find many products at affordable prices in stores or online. Beyond the basics like a can opener, spatula, and whisk, you will need:

Baking sheets: A necessity for baking and roasting. These are used in many savory and sweet recipes.

Blender or food processor: These are great to have on hand to help chop, blend, puree, and mix things together. You can also use them to create different types of flours to make cooking simpler.

Cake pans: Despite its name, a cake pan isn't just for baking cakes. It can be used to make casseroles and lasagnas as well. I suggest having a square one (9-by-9 inch) and a rectangular one (13-by-9 inch).

Colander: This tool is used for draining pasta and rice; I also use it for washing and draining fruits and vegetables.

Cooking pans or skillets: Cast iron, nonstick, or stainless steel are great options for cookware. You will want to have at least two different sizes, one medium (10-inch) and one large (12-inch). These are used for searing, sautéing, and frying.

Cutting board: This is used for chopping fruits, vegetables, and meats. I prefer color-coded ones so that I avoid any cross contamination with raw meats and fresh fruits and vegetables.

Knife set: A good-quality knife set is important to have in every kitchen. Knife sets can be pricey, but you can get away with just having a chef's knife. However, I recommend starting out with at least three knives: a chef's knife, a paring knife, and a serrated knife.

Measuring cups and spoons: These are used to measure out ingredients in recipes, but are also useful for portioning out foods to ensure you are staying within your nutrient goals and not over- or undereating.

Measuring scale: A food scale is needed to measure and portion your food more precisely. These can typically measure in grams and ounces. You'll notice the recipes include precise measurements for many ingredients, so investing in a scale is paramount for those with CKD.

Mixing bowls: These are important to help you prepare your ingredients. I prefer to buy the nested versions to save space and have a wide variety of sizes to work with.

Peeler: These are easy to use for peeling fruits and vegetables. While I typically encourage clients to keep peels and skins on fruits and veggies for extra fiber and nutrients, some recipes require you to remove them.

Saucepan: A smaller 3-quart saucepan is great for making sauces and when you don't necessarily need to make large quantities of food.

Stock or soup pot: A 6-quart pot is a good size to have. You can use stock or soup pots to make soups, stews, and stocks, boil pasta or rice, and cook many one-pot meals.

Nice-to-Have Kitchen Tools

Air fryer: An air fryer is similar to a convection oven; it uses hot air on rapid circulation to cook food quickly and make it crispy. It is super easy to clean up as well. An air fryer can cook almost anything, and it prepares food in a way that uses less fat than traditional frying methods.

Mandoline: This easy to use and affordable tool is great to have to make chopping, slicing, and grating easier. It also can help with making food more eye-catching, since you can slice things uniformly for better presentation.

Multifunction cooker: This tool can act as a pressure cooker, sauté pan, steamer, slow cooker, and an air fryer. This is useful for smaller kitchens, because you can just have one appliance on your counter versus five different ones.

Pressure cooker or slow cooker: Pressure cookers can cook food quickly, usually in less than half the time it would take on the stove or in the oven. Slow cookers cook foods slowly on lower heat and are great for busy days as well. You can toss all your ingredients in, leave the cooker to do its thing, and your meal can be ready when you return.

But What Should I Eat?

As I mentioned before, there is no one-size-fits-all approach to nutrition with CKD. Every person will have different needs and restrictions. Depending on your specific needs, you may want to keep those charts from chapter 1 handy to ensure that you are staying within your nutrient goals. While the renal diet may seem complicated, knowing what you can and can't eat is crucial for your success.

Foods to Enjoy

Fruits and vegetables: Eating a variety of colorful fruits and vegetables will provide you with a balanced number of vitamins, minerals, and antioxidants. Unless you need to restrict potassium (see page 12), all fruits and vegetables, fresh and frozen, can be part of a healthy diet.

Whole grains: Whole-grain foods are high in nutrients, packed with fiber, and can help combat many health conditions such as CKD, diabetes, and heart disease. Try to make half of your grain intake whole grains, which include amaranth; barley; brown and wild rice; buckwheat; oatmeal; popcorn; quinoa; and whole-grain breads, tortillas, and crackers.

Plant-based proteins: These types of proteins are easier on your kidneys and provide you with essential nutrients and fiber and include beans and legumes, nuts and seeds, soy, tempeh, and tofu. Dried, canned, or fresh are all great options but be mindful of sodium content and try to choose those that are low-sodium or no-salt-added.

Other: Coffee, tea, water, and unsweetened beverages; eggs; olive and avocado oils and vinegar; and spices and seasonings are also included in a healthy renal diet.

Foods to Limit or Avoid

The following foods should be avoided or at least limited to being consumed less than once a week.

Animal proteins: Though these types of proteins are considered high nutritional value, they are more taxing on your kidneys to metabolize and produce more wastes. It is best to limit your intake of animal proteins like beef, pork, poultry, and lamb, to less than once per week to protect your kidneys. For fish and seafood, limit intake to two times or less per week.

Highly processed, convenience foods: These types of foods are often packed with added sodium, sugars, and additives that can be hard on the kidneys.

- Food with saturated fats (bacon fat, margarine)
- High-sodium processed meats (bacon, bologna, pastrami, corned beef, hot dogs)
- Pickles, olives, and relish
- Premade seasonings, sauces, dressings, and marinades
- Salty processed chips and snacks
- Sodium-rich canned foods (sauces, marinades, soups)

Foods with added sugars: It is recommended that adults limit their added sugar intake to less than 10 percent of total calorie intake. Added sugar is not to be confused with sugar that naturally occurs in foods such as fruits. Added sugars are those that are put in foods during processing. Eating too much added sugar can increase your risk of heart disease and cause weight gain. Avoid dessert foods like ice cream, cookies, and candies, and juices and sodas (including diet sodas) on a renal diet.

Reading Nutrition Labels

Reading food labels is crucial to your success on the renal-friendly diet, because they give you key information that you need to keep track of your nutrient intake.

(A) **Serving Size:** Pay attention to how much is in a serving. The nutrition facts listed is per serving. Most people will eat more than 1 serving so it is important to know how much you are really consuming.

(B) **Calories:** The number of calories is listed per serving.

(C) **Sodium:** Most people with CKD will want to control their intake of sodium. Try to find products with less than 5 percent DV of sodium, less than 140 mg, or a sodium amount that is less than the number of calories.

(D) **Carbohydrates:** If you are diabetic and need to control your carbohydrate intake, pay close attention to the total carbohydrates listed on the label. Most people will only look at the total sugars, but all carbohydrates break down into sugar in your body.

(E) **Protein:** The CKD stage you are at will determine what your protein goals are. Be mindful of this number if you are on a low-protein diet.

Nutrition Facts	
Serving Size 1 Cup	
Servings Per Container 5	
Amount Per Serving	
Calories	**310**
	% Daily Value
Total Fat 4g	**5%**
Saturated Fat 0g	**0%**
Trans Fat 0g	**0%**
Cholesterol 0mg	**0%**
Sodium 200mg	**10%**
Total Carbohydrate 36g	**15%**
Dietary Fiber 5g	**17%**
Total Sugars 13g	**13%**
Includes 10g Added Sugars	**20%**
Protein 10g	
Vitamin D 4mcg	
Calcium 227mg	
Iron 8mg	
Potassium 159mg	

(F) **Potassium:** This nutrient has recently been added as a required listing on the nutrition facts label. If you need to limit your intake, then pay close attention to what is listed.

Phosphorus: This is not required to be on a food label. However, if you need to control your phosphorus intake, then you will want to pay attention to the ingredients list on the food package and look for phosphate additives. Look for words that contain "phos" in them, such as monocalcium phosphate, phosphoric acid, and trisodium phosphate.

Different brands of products will have varying nutrition profiles due to differences in ingredients. When choosing between products, remember to read food labels and compare to choose the best item for you and your dietary needs.

Cooking (and Eating) In the Real World

Now that you have a good understanding of the renal diet, it's time to learn how to apply these guidelines in the real world. I can give you all the information you want, but it's how you apply it to your life that will be the key to your success. In the real world, you won't always be eating at home; there will be times when you have family or social gatherings, work functions, or you simply just want to enjoy a meal dining out. These are all okay, and I encourage you to enjoy these events while still keeping in mind your dietary needs.

Cooking for the Whole Family

Many of the recipes in this book can appeal to all members of the family. What I find is the most difficult for most families to adapt to is the decrease in sodium. The best way to make sure all family members can enjoy the same foods is by offering different ways to customize with a toppings bar. Allow others to add more salt, herbs and seasonings of their choice, scallions, sour cream or Greek yogurt, sauces, etc. to their food.

The protein portions of the recipes are likely lower than what most family members need, but this can be easily remedied by cooking more protein for other members of the family.

Three Strategies for Eating Out

Dining out can still be an enjoyable experience while following a CKD-friendly diet. It's important for you to fully understand your diet, so that you can make conscious choices when eating out and continue to stick to your diet.

1. **If possible, plan ahead.** Before heading to or while you are waiting at the restaurant, look up the menu so that you are aware of what is available and what you can have on your diet. Don't be afraid to ask questions—you may want to know how something is prepared, what it is cooked in, or what sauces are used.

2. **Pay attention to protein portions.** The typical restaurant portions for all macronutrients are usually more than the average person needs. Be sure to portion out your food prior to eating to avoid going over your daily allowances. Try sharing a meal with someone else or packing up the extra before digging in.

3. **Order a la carte.** Sometimes it's better to order items a la carte instead of as a meal, since these are usually served without extra sauces or seasonings. You can also ask for sauces or dressings on the side and request that no salt be added to your meal.

If you have any questions, be sure to talk to your dietitian. They should be able to help further guide you and individualize your specific dining-out needs.

Handling Slipups

Sometimes you might get carried away by the enjoyment of eating out with family, friends, or colleagues, or maybe you just indulged a little bit too much. One little slipup isn't going to make everything come crashing down. What's important is that on most days, you are sticking to your diet. Don't overwhelm yourself with guilt or worry; instead, just get back on track at the next meal or snack. Remember to give yourself some grace, as this diet can be overwhelming and sometimes you might not be able to stick to it 100 percent.

About the Recipes

The recipes in this book are designed to make the renal diet easy by providing you with quick, simple, and delicious meals that lean on affordable and accessible ingredients. Most of the recipes are appropriate for all stages of CKD. For those with advanced CKD (stage 4 or 5), many of the recipes can be modified or adjusted; however, the nutritional needs of those with advanced CKD are very specific and must be tailored to the individual. Consult with your renal dietitian for a personal plan of care.

The recipes are categorized by type, and each recipe is labeled according to its nutrient content and/or ease of cooking.

→   Each recipe has been labeled as **High-**, **Medium-**, or **Low-Protein**. Your stage of CKD and protein needs will determine which recipes you can try. Those with a higher stage, such as stage 4 or 5, may want to stick with the Low-Protein recipes. However, many recipes include tips on how you can adjust the recipe to better fit your needs.

→   Some recipes are labeled as **Diabetes-Friendly** and/or **Heart-Healthy**. These are appropriate for those with diabetes or hypertension. There are also tips throughout the recipes that show you how to make something Diabetes-Friendly or Heart-Healthy.

→   There are also some recipes that use **5 Ingredients or Fewer** (excluding salt, pepper, and oil). These are generally recipes that will be quick to make and easy breezy.

→   Some recipes are **One Pot** meals, which means they can be made in one single cooking vessel. This makes cleanup a breeze, because who enjoys washing dishes?

Finally, each recipe includes nutrition facts per serving. All nutrients are rounded to the nearest whole number, except for protein. Protein is a macronutrient that you want to be extra mindful of when eating a renal-friendly diet to help protect your kidneys. There are also tips included throughout the recipes if you need to make particular adjustments for protein, potassium, phosphorus, diabetes, or hypertension, or to make recipes even easier.

The 7-Day Kickstarter Meal Plan

Now that I have provided you with the basic information on a kidney-friendly diet, it's time for you to start planning. I've included a weeklong sample meal plan to help you get started.

This meal plan is to serve as a guide; your needs will be different based on nutrition status, stage of CKD, and any other comorbidities you may have. This plan is flexible, and you can adjust accordingly based on your needs as well as your food preferences.

This meal plan serves one person and makes use of leftovers throughout the week so you aren't cooking every day or left with food waste. (Remember to always allow food to cool completely, and to label and date leftovers before storing in the freezer.) If you need more food throughout the week, feel free to include fruit, snacks from chapter 7, or add a salad or soup from chapter 4 to your lunch or dinner.

Start the Week Right

Plan ahead to make sure you are equipped to prepare your meals for the week to come. Refer to your nutrient tracker from chapter 1 to make sure you are sticking to your daily nutrient allowances. Review and choose recipes beforehand, check your pantry for what ingredients you have, and use a shopping list so that you are sticking to your plan.

The Mango Teriyaki Sauce (page 140) can be made at the beginning of the week and kept in your refrigerator for quick and easy access. The Tangy Lemon Energy Bites (page 123) can also be made ahead and kept in the freezer until ready to eat. Wash and prep any ingredients ahead of time so you can quickly access them when ready to cook.

Some recipes may seem to have a lot of ingredients, but you will find that most are spices and seasonings to flavor the dish. Furthermore, the shopping list for this week may seem long, but you likely already have many of the ingredients. If not, you will also find that many of the following ingredients are pantry staples and can be stored and used across a wide variety of recipes.

Don't feel overwhelmed—eating should be an enjoyable and nourishing experience!

	BREAKFAST	LUNCH	DINNER	SNACKS	TOTAL NUTRIENTS
SUN	· Plant-Powered Breakfast Wrap (page 53) · Cinnamon Hazelnut Latte (page 42)	· Feta, Onion, and Pepper Pizza (page 88) · 1 cup fresh strawberries	· Spicy Black Bean Power Bowl (page 81)	· 6 Glutino yogurt-covered pretzels · 7 Flavis low-protein crackers + ½ cup olives + 1 tablespoon cottage cheese	· 1,570 calories · 41.8g protein · 1,840mg sodium · 1,710mg potassium · 530mg phosphorus
MON	· *Leftover* Plant-Powered Breakfast Wrap · 6 ounces black coffee · 1 medium pear	· *Leftover* Feta, Onion, and Pepper Pizza · 6 Glutino yogurt-covered pretzels	· Roasted Vegetable and Tofu Fried Rice (page 76)	· Tangy Lemon Energy Bite (page 123) · 1 small apple + 1 tablespoon unsalted nut butter	· 1,550 calories · 42.9g protein · 1,140mg sodium · 1,620mg potassium · 560mg phosphorus
TUES	· Chocolate Coconut Pancakes (page 48) · 6 ounces black coffee · 1 cup fresh strawberries	· *Leftover* Spicy Black Bean Power Bowl · *Leftover* Tangy Lemon Energy Bite	· *Leftover* Feta, Onion, and Pepper Pizza	· Cinnamon Apple Chia Seed Pudding (page 125)	· 1,430 calories · 36.9g protein · 1,000mg sodium · 1,775mg potassium · 875mg phosphorus
WED	· *Leftover* Plant-Powered Breakfast Wrap · *Leftover* Cinnamon Hazelnut Latte	· *Leftover* Spicy Black Bean Power Bowl · *Leftover* Tangy Lemon Energy Bite	· *Leftover* Feta, Onion, and Pepper Pizza	· 1 small apple + 1 tablespoon unsalted nut butter · 7 Flavis low-protein crackers + ½ cup olives + 1 tablespoon cottage cheese	· 1,660 calories · 45.7g protein · 1,590mg sodium · 1,880mg potassium · 630mg phosphorus

CONTINUED ▶

	BREAKFAST	LUNCH	DINNER	SNACKS	TOTAL NUTRIENTS
THURS	· *Leftover* Plant-Powered Breakfast Wrap · *Leftover* Cinnamon Hazelnut Latte	· *Leftover* Roasted Vegetable and Tofu Fried Rice · 8 Flavis low-protein shortbread cookies	· *Leftover* Spicy Black Bean Power Bowl · 6 Glutino yogurt-covered pretzels	· *Leftover* Tangy Lemon Energy Bite · 1 small apple + 1 tablespoon unsalted nut butter	· 1,690 calories · 45.5g protein · 1,200mg sodium · 2,000mg potassium · 580mg phosphorus
FRI	· *Leftover* Chocolate Coconut Pancakes · 6 ounces black coffee · 1 medium pear	· *Leftover* Roasted Vegetable and Tofu Fried Rice · 8 Flavis low-protein shortbread cookies	· Sheet Pan Teriyaki Salmon with Roasted Vegetables (page 93)	· *Leftover* Tangy Lemon Energy Bite · 7 Flavis low-protein crackers + ½ cup olives + 1 tablespoon cottage cheese	· 1,590 calories · 42.3g protein · 1,250mg sodium · 1,870mg potassium · 715mg phosphorus
SAT	· *Leftover* Chocolate Coconut Pancakes · 1 cup fresh strawberries	· *Leftover* Roasted Vegetable and Tofu Fried Rice · 8 Flavis low-protein shortbread cookies	· *Leftover* Sheet Pan Teriyaki Salmon and Roasted Eggplant	· *Leftover* Tangy Lemon Energy Bite · 7 Flavis low-protein crackers + ½ cup olives + 1 tablespoon cottage cheese	· 1,530 calories · 42.7g protein · 1,230 mg sodium · 1,900mg potassium · 730mg phosphorus

Meal plan based on a 5-foot, 2-inch woman, weighing 110 pounds with Diabetes and Stage 3 CKD.

Shopping List

FRESH AND FROZEN PRODUCE

- Apples, small (4)
- Basil (1 bunch) (optional)
- Bell peppers, red (5)
- Carrot, medium (1)
- Cauliflower rice, frozen, 1 (10-ounce) bag
- Eggplant, medium (2)
- Garlic (1 head)
- Ginger (1-inch piece)
- Lemon (1)
- Mango (1)
- Medjool dates, pitted (8)
- Mustard greens (4 cups)
- Onion, white, small (1)
- Pears (2)
- Red onion, small (1)
- Strawberries (3 cups)
- Sweet potato, medium (1)
- Turnip, medium (1)
- Zucchini (1)

PANTRY

- Avocado or olive oil
- Avocado or olive oil cooking spray
- Baking powder
- Black pepper, ground
- Brown rice
- Brown sugar, light
- Cashews, unsalted
- Cayenne pepper, ground
- Cinnamon, ground
- Chia seeds
- Cocoa powder, unsweetened
- Coconut aminos or low-sodium soy sauce
- Coconut, shredded, unsweetened
- Coffee, ground
- Cumin, ground
- Flour, all-purpose
- Flour, whole-wheat
- Garlic powder
- Ginger, ground
- Italian seasoning
- Maple syrup
- Nut butter, unsalted
- Nutritional yeast
- Olives
- Rice vinegar
- Sesame oil
- Siete brand hot sauce
- Sugar, granulated
- Torani Sugar-Free Classic Hazelnut Syrup
- Turmeric, ground
- Vanilla extract
- Yeast, active dry

CONTINUED ▶

CANNED, JARRED, BAGGED, AND BOTTLED ITEMS

- Black beans, no-salt-added or low-sodium, 1 (15-ounce) can
- Chickpeas, low-sodium or no-salt-added, 2 (15-ounce) cans
- Coconut milk, lite unsweetened, 1 (13.5-ounce) can
- Flavis Fette Tostate low-protein crackers, 1 (7.2-ounce) package
- Flavis Frollini low-protein shortbread cookies, 1 (7.1-ounce) package
- Glutino yogurt-covered pretzels, 1 (5.5-ounce) package
- Pico de gallo or salsa, low-sodium, 1 (16-ounce) container
- Whole-grain tortillas, 4 (10-inch)

EGGS, DAIRY, AND DAIRY ALTERNATIVES

- Almond milk, plain unsweetened (1 quart)
- Cottage cheese, low-fat (¼ cup)
- Eggs, large (3)
- Feta cheese (6 ounces)
- Half-and-half (4 ounces)

MEAT, POULTRY, SEAFOOD, AND PLANT PROTEINS

- Salmon, wild-caught, 1 (4-ounce) fillet
- Tofu, firm, 1 (14-ounce) package

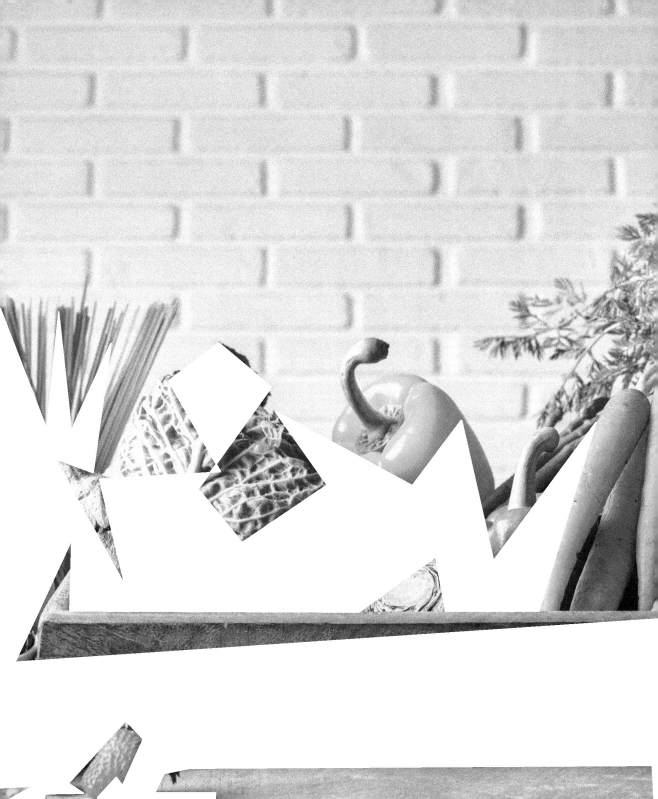

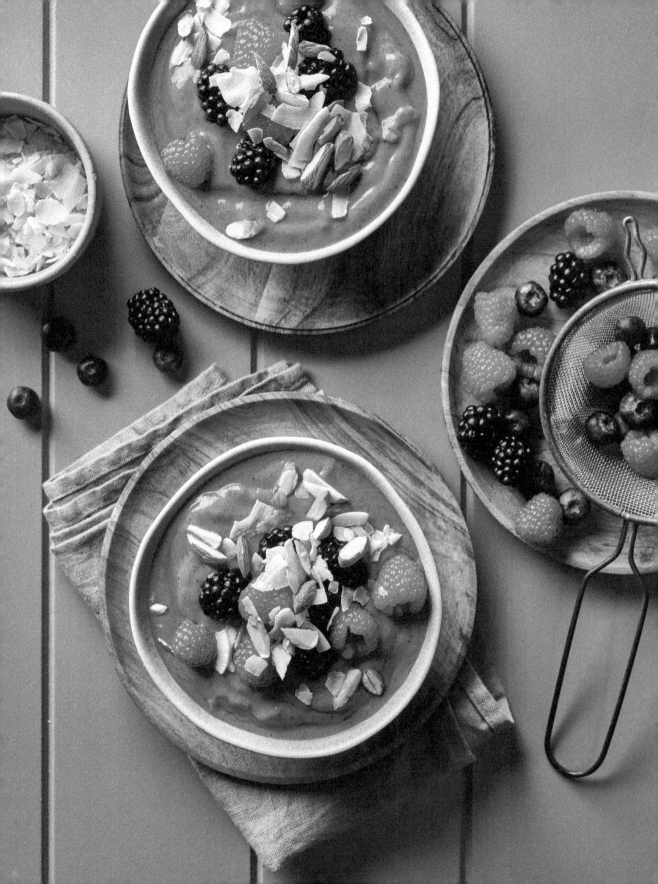

3

Beverages and Breakfast

◁ Acai Berry Smoothie Bowls, page 45

Cinnamon Hazelnut Latte

DIABETES-FRIENDLY • LOW-PROTEIN • 5 INGREDIENTS OR FEWER

SERVES 5 • PREP TIME: 10 minutes

Coffee can be a part of a healthy diet when consumed in moderation (about 1 cup per day). Coffee contains antioxidants, is anti-inflammatory, and is anti-carcinogenic, but be careful when drinking coffee beverages with excess amounts of added sugars and flavorings. Customize this drink by trying other flavors (such as vanilla or mocha) and switching up the liquid (try oat milk or coconut milk). Pair with an Oatmeal Breakfast Cookie (page 46) or some Chocolate Coconut Pancakes (page 48).

1 cup plain Unsweetened Almond Milk (page 143) or store-bought

½ cup half-and-half

4 cups brewed coffee

10 teaspoons Torani Sugar-Free Classic Hazelnut Syrup

5 cinnamon sticks or 5 dashes ground cinnamon

1. In a large pitcher, combine the almond milk and half-and-half and whisk until combined.

2. Add the coffee and stir until combined.

3. Add 2 teaspoons of hazelnut syrup to each mug. Divide the coffee mixture evenly into the 5 mugs.

4. Garnish each mug with a cinnamon stick or a dash of ground cinnamon and enjoy!

5. Store leftovers in an airtight container in the refrigerator for up to 3 days.

MAKE IT HEART-HEALTHY: Leave out the half-and-half and use more unsweetened almond milk.

PER SERVING (1 CUP): Calories: 20; Protein: 1.2g; Carbohydrates: 3g; Fiber 2g; Total Fat: 1g; Saturated Fat: 0g; Sodium: 68mg; Cholesterol: 0mg; Potassium: 284mg; Phosphorus: 13mg

Chai Tea Latte

DIABETES-FRIENDLY • HEART-HEALTHY • LOW-PROTEIN • ONE POT

SERVES 2 • **PREP TIME:** 2 minutes • **COOK TIME:** 15 minutes

Tea contains less caffeine than coffee and is a great alternative to start your day with. This recipe is the perfect blend of creaminess and spice, and pairs well with PB&J Overnight Oats (page 47) or Egg-Stuffed Avocado (page 51). For a caffeine-free version, leave out the tea bags and just add the spices to warmed milk.

1½ cups plain Unsweetened Almond Milk (page 143) or store-bought

½ cup half-and-half

2 black tea bags

2 tablespoons maple syrup

¾ teaspoon ground cinnamon

¼ teaspoon ground ginger

⅛ teaspoon ground cloves

1. In a small saucepan, combine the almond milk and half-and-half.

2. Heat the mixture over medium-low heat for about 5 minutes, or until the milk begins to bubble around the edges of the pan. Stir occasionally to prevent the milk from scalding.

3. Turn off the heat and add the tea bags to the milk. Steep the tea for 3 to 5 minutes, or to your preferred strength. Remove the tea bags after steeping.

4. Add the maple syrup, cinnamon, ginger, and cloves to the saucepan. Turn the heat to medium and whisk for 2 to 3 minutes, until the mixture is combined and the tea is hot and starting to steam.

5. Divide between cups. Adjust the flavorings and sweetness to taste. Serve hot or over ice.

6. You can double the recipe and store leftovers in an airtight container in the refrigerator for up to 4 days.

PER SERVING (1 CUP): Calories: 91; Protein: 2.2g; Carbohydrates: 17g; Fiber 2g; Total Fat: 2g; Saturated Fat: 0g; Sodium: 166mg; Cholesterol: 0mg; Potassium: 446mg; Phosphorus: 17mg

Blueberry Cranberry Smoothie

HEART-HEALTHY • LOW-PROTEIN • ONE POT • 5 INGREDIENTS OR FEWER

SERVES 1 • **PREP TIME:** 5 minutes

Tofu is a plant-based protein with a mild flavor and gives this drink a smooth and creamy texture. This recipe uses unsweetened, plain cranberry juice, which gives it a bright and tart taste. You can use cranberry juice cocktail or an unsweetened plant-based milk to tone it down if you'd like.

¼ cup unsweetened plain cranberry juice, plus more as needed

1 cup frozen blueberries

½ cup silken tofu

1 teaspoon vanilla extract

½ cup ice (optional)

1. Pour the cranberry juice into a blender.

2. Add the blueberries, tofu, and vanilla and blend until very smooth. Add the ice for a thicker consistency or more liquid for a thinner consistency.

3. Serve immediately.

MAKE IT DIABETES-FRIENDLY: Substitute the juice with an unsweetened plain plant-based milk such as oat or almond to lower the carbohydrate content, or add protein powder to increase the protein content depending on your needs. Note: Protein content varies among different brands, so be sure to check your nutrition label.

PER SERVING: Calories: 224; Protein: 9.5g; Carbohydrates: 36g; Fiber 6g; Total Fat: 5g; Saturated Fat: 1g; Sodium: 55mg; Cholesterol: 0mg; Potassium: 411mg; Phosphorus: 137mg

Acai Berry Smoothie Bowls

DIABETES-FRIENDLY • HEART-HEALTHY • MEDIUM-PROTEIN • ONE POT

SERVES 2 • PREP TIME: 10 minutes

Acai (pronounced ah-sigh-EE) is a fruit harvested from the rain forests of South America. Acai berries are considered a "superfood" and are high in antioxidants and fiber. An easy way to incorporate this fruit into your diet is with a refreshing smoothie bowl. You can find acai packets in the frozen fruit section of most grocery store retailers. Customize the bowl by swapping out different fruits and toppings, or toast the shredded coconut flakes if desired.

1 (14-ounce) packet unsweetened frozen acai

1 cup unsweetened frozen berries (mixed berries, strawberries, blueberries, or raspberries)

½ cup plain nonfat or low-fat Greek yogurt

¼ to ½ cup unsweetened plain rice milk (depending on your thickness preference)

¼ medium apple or pear

1 tablespoon blackberries

1 tablespoon raspberries

1 tablespoon sliced almonds

1 tablespoon unsweetened shredded coconut

1. Empty the unsweetened frozen acai packet into a blender. If the product is one big pureed block, break it into small pieces.

2. Add the frozen berries, yogurt, ¼ cup of rice milk, and the apple into the blender. Blend until smooth. The consistency should be thick. Add more liquid if needed to reach the desired consistency.

3. Divide the blended mixture evenly between bowls. Top each bowl with ½ tablespoon each of the blackberries, raspberries, almonds, and coconut. Enjoy.

MAKE IT LOWER IN PROTEIN AND POTASSIUM: You can lower the protein and potassium content of this recipe by leaving out the yogurt. Add more liquid as needed to reach the desired consistency.

PER SERVING (1 BOWL): Calories: 281; Protein: 14.6g; Carbohydrates: 36g; Fiber: 4g; Total Fat: 9g; Saturated Fat: 2g; Sodium: 146mg; Cholesterol: 11mg; Potassium: 353mg; Phosphorus: 173mg

Oatmeal Breakfast Cookies

DIABETES-FRIENDLY • HEART-HEALTHY • LOW-PROTEIN

MAKES 14 COOKIES • **PREP TIME:** 10 minutes • **COOK TIME:** 15 minutes

Who says you can't have cookies for breakfast? This tasty breakfast cookie is jam-packed with healthy fats and B vitamins and is great for busy mornings or when you are craving a snack. These can also be made ahead and stored in the freezer. When buying maple syrup and nut butter, be sure to read the ingredients list and choose a pure product without added sugars or flavorings.

2 cups quick oats

1 cup creamy unsalted nut butter of choice

½ cup chopped walnuts

⅓ cup unsweetened dried cranberries

¼ cup pumpkin puree

¼ cup maple syrup

3 tablespoons ground flaxseed

1 teaspoon ground cinnamon

½ teaspoon salt

MAKE IT SIMPLER: If you don't have quick oats, make your own. Pour 2 cups of rolled oats into a blender and pulse a few times to break them down.

1. Preheat the oven to 325°F. Line a large baking sheet with parchment paper or a silicone baking mat and set aside.

2. In a stand mixer using a paddle attachment or in a large bowl, combine the oats, nut butter, walnuts, cranberries, pumpkin puree, maple syrup, flaxseed, cinnamon, and salt. Mix until the dough comes together.

3. Using a large ice-cream scoop, tightly pack the dough into the scoop. Drop the batter onto the prepared baking sheet and flatten slightly. The cookies will not spread but be sure to keep them evenly spaced on the sheet.

4. Bake for 15 minutes, or until slightly browned. Remove from the oven and cool completely.

5. Store leftovers in an airtight container for up to 6 days, or in the freezer for up to 3 months.

PER SERVING (1 COOKIE): Calories: 214; Protein: 6.3g; Carbohydrates: 19g; Fiber: 4g; Total Fat: 14g; Saturated Fat: 1g; Sodium: 91mg; Cholesterol: 0mg; Potassium: 207mg; Phosphorus: 153mg

PB&J Overnight Oats

DIABETES-FRIENDLY • HEART-HEALTHY • LOW-PROTEIN • ONE POT

SERVES 1 • **PREP TIME:** 5 minutes, plus 8 hours or overnight to chill

Overnight oats can make mornings a breeze. They are simple to put together the night before and there are tons of different flavor combinations you can try. Start with a base of rolled oats, add your choice of plain unsweetened milk, and vary the toppings: Try other fruits, cacao nibs, various nut or sunflower seed butters, and different spices. For a little bit of sweetness, add ¼ teaspoon of maple syrup or honey. Trader Joe's has a great peanut butter product made from unsalted dry-roasted peanuts with no sodium and no sugar added. Be sure to read the food labels to ensure no added ingredients to keep it healthy.

½ cup plain Unsweetened Almond Milk (page 143) or store-bought

⅓ cup rolled oats

¼ cup frozen strawberries

1 tablespoon unsalted peanut butter

1 teaspoon vanilla extract

Dash ground cinnamon

1. In a small bowl or 8-ounce mason jar, combine the almond milk, oats, strawberries, peanut butter, vanilla, and cinnamon and mix together.

2. Cover and refrigerate overnight or for at least 8 hours.

3. When ready to enjoy, stir again and mash up the strawberries. Or, if desired, warm in the microwave for about 1 minute.

PER SERVING: Calories: 245; Protein: 7.8g; Carbohydrates: 28g; Fiber: 6g; Total Fat: 11g; Saturated Fat: 2g; Sodium: 68mg; Cholesterol: 0mg; Potassium: 272mg; Phosphorus: 118mg

Chocolate Coconut Pancakes

DIABETES-FRIENDLY • LOW-PROTEIN

SERVES 4 • **PREP TIME:** 15 minutes • **COOK TIME:** 15 minutes

Cocoa powder is made from crushed cocoa beans that has the fat (aka the cocoa butter) portion of the bean removed. It is rich in antioxidants, which help with reducing inflammation, improving cholesterol and increasing brain function. When choosing maple syrup, pay attention to the label and ingredients list to ensure a pure product that is made from maple syrup and not just maple flavoring or something with added sugars.

1 cup whole-wheat flour

2 tablespoons granulated sugar

1 tablespoon baking powder

1 tablespoon unsweetened cocoa powder

⅔ cup unsweetened lite canned coconut milk

¼ to ½ cup water

1 large egg

1 teaspoon avocado oil

½ teaspoon vanilla extract

Avocado or olive oil cooking spray

2 tablespoons maple syrup

¼ cup unsweetened coconut flakes

1 tablespoon raspberries or strawberries, for topping (optional)

1. In a large mixing bowl, mix the flour, sugar, baking powder, and cocoa powder.

2. In a medium mixing bowl, mix together coconut milk, ¼ cup of water, the egg, avocado oil, and vanilla.

3. Pour the wet mixture into the dry mixture and slowly fold together until the batter is wet. Add more water, up to ¼ cup, if needed. Be careful not to overmix.

4. Heat a medium pan or griddle over medium heat. Spray the pan with a little bit of cooking spray.

5. Spoon about 2 tablespoons of batter onto the pan to form 4-inch pancakes. Cook for 3 to 5 minutes, and flip when you start to see bubbling. Cook for another 3 minutes. Repeat with the remaining batter.

6. Top each pancake with a drizzle of maple syrup and a sprinkle of coconut flakes and any optional ingredients (if using). Serve immediately and enjoy!

1 teaspoon choco-
late chips, for topping
(optional)

Powdered sugar, for
topping (optional)

7. Store leftovers in an airtight container or resealable
bag in the refrigerator for up to 3 days. If freezing,
layer parchment paper between the pancakes. Store
in an airtight container or resealable bag in the
freezer for up to 3 months. When ready to eat, pop
the pancakes into the toaster oven at 300°F for
15 minutes to reheat.

MAKE IT HEART-HEALTHY: Substitute the canned
coconut milk with a plant-based milk of your choice.
Try almond, rice, or oat milk, or try making your own
Unsweetened Almond Milk (page 143).

PER SERVING (3 PANCAKES): Calories: 246; Protein: 6.2g;
Carbohydrates: 40g; Fiber: 5g; Total Fat: 9g; Saturated Fat: 5g;
Sodium: 399mg; Cholesterol: 47mg; Potassium: 195mg;
Phosphorus: 225mg

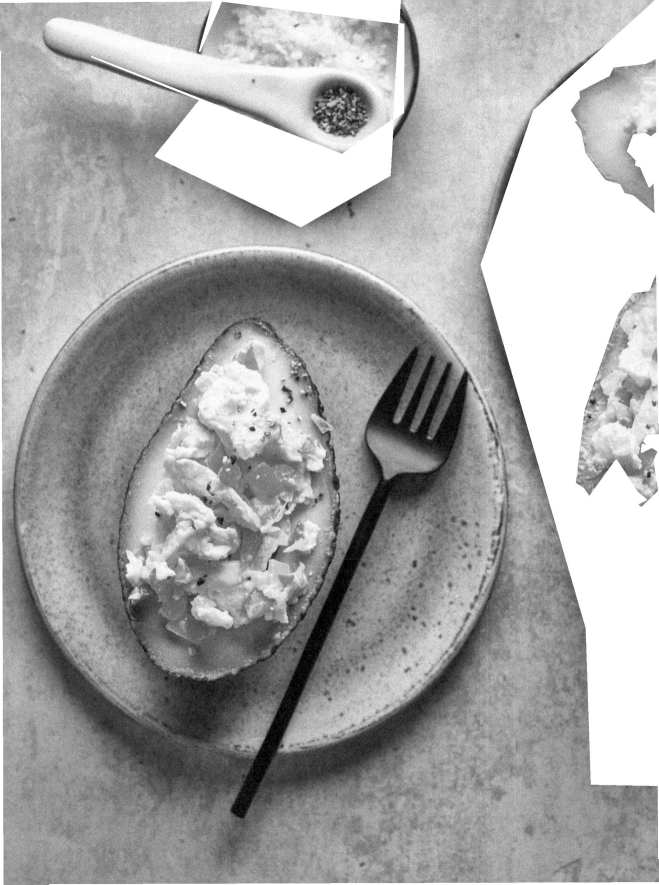

Egg-Stuffed Avocado

DIABETES-FRIENDLY • LOW-PROTEIN • ONE POT • 5 INGREDIENTS OR FEWER

SERVES 1 • **PREP TIME:** 10 minutes • **COOK TIME:** 10 minutes

Avocadoes are loaded with vitamins and minerals as well as fiber and healthy fats. This meal will leave you feeling full and satisfied, and can be made ahead and stored in the refrigerator. Enjoy it cold or hot by popping it in the oven at 300°F for 5 minutes.

1 teaspoon olive or avocado oil

¼ cup chopped red bell pepper

¼ cup chopped yellow onion

1 large egg, beaten

½ avocado, pitted

Pinch freshly ground black pepper

Pinch salt

Lemon zest, for topping (about 1 teaspoon) (optional)

1. In a medium nonstick skillet, heat the oil over medium heat.

2. Add the bell pepper and onion to the pan and cook for about 3 minutes, until softened and the onions are slightly translucent.

3. Move the veggies over to one side of the pan. Add the egg to the other side of the pan and stir gently until set.

4. Gently fold the veggies into the scrambled eggs. Remove from the heat and spoon the scrambled egg mixture into the avocado cavity. Season with a pinch of salt and black pepper.

5. Add some lemon zest (if using) on top to brighten up the recipe and add some pizzazz!

MAKE IT HEART-HEALTHY: Lower the sodium content by omitting the salt. Instead, use your favorite herbs and spices (try basil, thyme, or rosemary) to add some flavor.

MAKE IT LOWER IN POTASSIUM: Swap out the avocado for a bell pepper. Using a bell pepper as your boat will lower this by 100 calories and 241mg potassium.

PER SERVING: Calories: 264; Protein: 8.7g; Carbohydrates: 14g; Fiber: 6g; Total Fat: 21g; Saturated Fat: 4g; Sodium: 225mg; Cholesterol: 187mg; Potassium: 553mg; Phosphorus: 147mg

Loaded Veggie Egg Cups with Toast

DIABETES-FRIENDLY • HEART-HEALTHY • MEDIUM-PROTEIN

SERVES 4 • PREP TIME: 15 minutes **• COOK TIME:** 25 minutes

This is a breakfast you can make ahead of time and store in the refrigerator or freezer for a grab-and-go morning option. Swap out the spices for any combination you enjoy. Try it with basil, dill, or parsley, or substitute with cayenne pepper and red pepper flakes for some spice.

1 tablespoon olive or avocado oil

½ cup shredded carrots

½ cup finely chopped yellow squash

½ cup finely chopped red or green bell pepper

½ cup finely chopped sweet onion

8 large eggs

1 tablespoon plain nonfat yogurt

1 teaspoon garlic powder

1 teaspoon ground turmeric

1 teaspoon freshly ground black pepper

Avocado or olive oil cooking spray

4 slices whole-wheat bread

1. Preheat the oven to 350°F.

2. In a medium skillet, heat the oil over medium heat. Add the carrots, squash, bell pepper, and onion and sauté for 3 to 5 minutes, until just softened. Remove from the pan and set aside to cool.

3. In a large bowl, whisk the eggs, yogurt, garlic powder, turmeric, and black pepper together. Add the cooled vegetables and mix together.

4. Spray a 12-cup muffin tin with cooking spray. Scoop the egg mixture evenly into the muffin tins. Bake for 20 to 25 minutes, or until the eggs have set in the middle. Meanwhile, toast your bread to the desired doneness. Serve.

5. Store leftovers in an airtight container in the refrigerator for up to 5 days or in the freezer for up to 3 months.

MAKE IT LOWER IN PHOSPHOROUS: Lower the phosphorus and cholesterol content by replacing 4 of the whole eggs with 6 egg whites or ¾ cup of liquid egg whites.

PER SERVING (3 EGG CUPS + 1 SLICE TOAST): Calories: 311; Protein: 18.5g; Carbohydrates: 24g; Fiber 4g; Total Fat: 16g; Saturated Fat: 4g; Sodium: 304mg; Cholesterol: 373mg; Potassium: 444mg; Phosphorus: 288mg

Plant-Powered Breakfast Wraps

DIABETES-FRIENDLY • HEART-HEALTHY • MEDIUM-PROTEIN

SERVES 4 • **PREP TIME:** 15 minutes • **COOK TIME:** 10 minutes

This is a great on-the-go breakfast wrap using chickpeas as the plant-powered protein source. You can even swap out the tortilla and have this as a breakfast bowl served over some brown rice or barley. Chickpeas are high in fiber, which is great for your gut health.

1 (15-ounce) can low-sodium or no-salt-added chickpeas

½ teaspoon ground turmeric

½ teaspoon freshly ground black pepper

2 teaspoons olive or avocado oil

½ medium white onion, finely chopped

½ red bell pepper, finely chopped

2 garlic cloves, minced

1 tablespoon nutritional yeast

4 (10-inch) whole-grain tortillas

4 teaspoons Siete brand hot sauce

1. Drain and rinse the chickpeas under running water, reserving 1 tablespoon of the liquid from the can.

2. In a medium bowl, combine the chickpeas and reserved chickpea liquid. Use a fork to gently mash the beans. Mix in the turmeric and black pepper until combined.

3. In a medium saucepan, heat the oil over medium heat. Add the onion, bell pepper, and garlic and sauté for 3 to 5 minutes until soft. Add the chickpea mixture and nutritional yeast and cook for 2 to 3 minutes, stirring occasionally until warm.

4. Meanwhile, warm the tortillas on a pan or in the oven for a few minutes. To assemble, divide the chickpea mixture into 4 equal portions and place on the tortillas. Top with hot sauce before wrapping.

5. These wraps can be stored in the freezer in an airtight container or freezer-safe resealable bag. When ready to eat again, heat in the oven at 350°F for 30 minutes.

PER SERVING (1 WRAP): Calories: 327; Protein: 12.8g; Carbohydrates: 50g; Fiber 12g; Total Fat: 9g; Saturated Fat: 2g; Sodium: 473mg; Cholesterol: 0mg; Potassium: 257mg; Phosphorus: 100mg

Tofu Breakfast Muffins

DIABETES-FRIENDLY • HEART-HEALTHY • MEDIUM-PROTEIN

SERVES 4 • PREP TIME: 15 minutes • **COOK TIME:** 30 minutes

Research shows that plant protein sources result in less kidney damage than animal proteins. These can be eaten hot, cold, on their own, or between a whole-wheat English muffin.

Avocado or olive oil cooking spray

16 ounces firm tofu, drained and patted dry

1 tablespoon, plus 2 teaspoons avocado oil

½ teaspoon salt

½ teaspoon ground turmeric

¼ teaspoon garlic powder

¼ teaspoon onion powder

¼ teaspoon ground cayenne pepper

2 tablespoons chickpea flour

8 ounces mushrooms, thinly sliced

1 medium red bell pepper, diced

2 tablespoons chopped shallot

MAKE IT SIMPLER: If you don't have chickpea flour, you can substitute it with ¼ cup of all-purpose flour.

1. Preheat the oven to 350°F. Spray a muffin tin with cooking spray.

2. In a food processor, combine the tofu, 1 tablespoon of avocado oil, the salt, turmeric, garlic powder, onion powder, and cayenne and process until smooth. Add the chickpea flour and process again until combined.

3. In a medium skillet or sauté pan, heat the remaining 2 teaspoons of avocado oil over medium heat and add the mushrooms. Cook for 5 minutes, or until the mushrooms have released some liquid and are starting to brown.

4. Add the bell pepper and shallot and cook for 5 minutes, until softened. Remove from the heat and add the vegetables to the tofu mixture in the food processor or blender.

5. Pulse 1 to 2 times until just combined. Don't over-pulse! Divide the mixture evenly into a greased muffin pan and bake for about 20 minutes, or until the muffins have set completely in the middle.

6. Store in an airtight container in the refrigerator for up to 5 days.

PER SERVING (3 MUFFINS): Calories: 225; Protein: 16.1g; Carbohydrates: 16g; Fiber 3g; Total Fat: 12g; Saturated Fat: 2g; Sodium: 316mg; Cholesterol: 0mg; Potassium: 500mg; Phosphorus: 250mg

Turkey Sausage Breakfast Casserole

DIABETES-FRIENDLY • MEDIUM-PROTEIN

SERVES 9 • **PREP TIME:** 15 minutes • **COOK TIME:** 1 hour 15 minutes

Using turkey sausage instead of beef or pork in this recipe helps cut down on extra fat and grease. Make this meal for Sunday family brunches or as an easy make-ahead meal since it stores well in the fridge.

8 ounces lean turkey sausage

8 ounces full-fat cream cheese

1 cup nonfat milk

3 large eggs

3 large egg whites or ½ cup liquid egg whites

1 tablespoon yellow mustard

½ teaspoon dried onion flakes

½ teaspoon garlic powder

¼ teaspoon freshly ground black pepper

Avocado or olive oil cooking spray

4 slices whole-wheat bread

MAKE IT HEART-HEALTHY: Use a low-fat or light cream cheese to lower the fat content.

1. Preheat the oven to 325°F.

2. In a medium skillet, crumble the sausage and cook over medium-high heat for 10 minutes, or until browned. Set aside.

3. Meanwhile, in a blender or food processor, combine the cream cheese, milk, eggs, egg whites, mustard, onion flakes, garlic powder, and pepper. Process until combined and smooth.

4. In a medium bowl, combine the cooked turkey sausage with the egg mixture and stir until combined.

5. Grease a 9-by-9-inch casserole or baking dish with cooking spray. Line the bottom of the pan with the bread. Pour the sausage and egg mixture over the bread. Bake for 55 minutes, or until the sausage and egg mixture is set. Divide into 9 equal portions and serve warm.

6. Store leftovers in an airtight container or resealable storage bag in the refrigerator for up to 5 days or in the freezer for up to 3 months.

PER SERVING (3-INCH SQUARE): Calories: 222; Protein: 12.3g; Carbohydrates: 12g; Fiber 1g; Fat: 14g; Saturated Fat: 6g; Sodium: 397mg; Cholesterol: 113mg; Potassium: 152mg; Phosphorus: 87mg

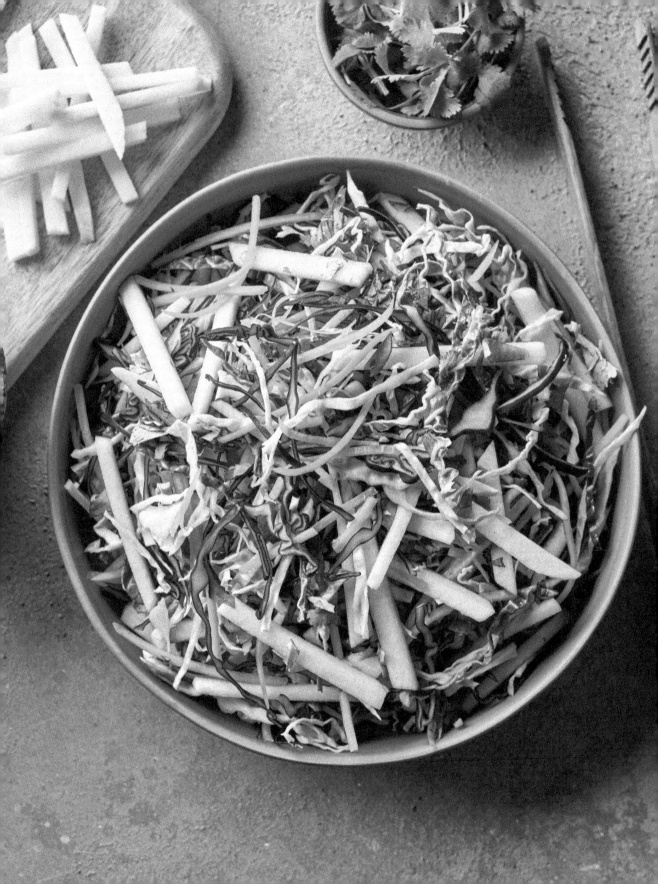

4
Salads, Vegetables, and Sides

◀ Jicama Cabbage Slaw, page 59

Crisp Cucumber Salad

DIABETES-FRIENDLY • HEART-HEALTHY • LOW-PROTEIN
ONE POT • 5 INGREDIENTS OR FEWER

SERVES 8 • PREP TIME: 10 minutes, plus 10 minutes to chill

Cucumber salads are cool, crisp, and refreshing. They work well as a kidney-friendly snack or as a side dish to a meal. I love that they are customizable with different types of vinegars and seasonings. Try white or apple cider vinegar and use your favorite herbs and spices to give this recipe a new twist. You can also toast the sesame seeds for an extra depth of flavor and omit the salt if desired.

4 large cucumbers, peeled to leave alternating green stripes

½ cup rice vinegar

2 teaspoons granulated sugar

¼ teaspoon salt

2 tablespoons sesame seeds

1. Cut the cucumbers in half lengthwise and scrape out the seeds with a spoon.

2. Using a sharp kitchen knife, vegetable peeler, or mandoline, cut the cucumbers into paper-thin slices. You can increase the thickness if you prefer.

3. Put the cucumber slices on a paper towel and squeeze gently to remove any excess liquid.

4. In a small bowl, combine the rice vinegar, sugar, and salt and stir until the sugar and salt have dissolved.

5. Add the cucumbers and sesame seeds to the vinegar mixture and stir until combined. You can serve immediately or let marinate for 10 minutes for more flavor infusion.

6. Store leftovers in an airtight container in the refrigerator for up to 5 days.

PER SERVING (1 CUP): Calories: 38; Protein: 1g; Carbohydrates: 5g; Fiber: 2g; Total Fat: 2g; Saturated Fat: 0g; Sodium: 77mg; Cholesterol: 0mg; Potassium: 168mg; Phosphorus: 42mg

Jicama Cabbage Slaw

DIABETES-FRIENDLY • HEART-HEALTHY • LOW-PROTEIN

SERVES 8 • PREP TIME: 20 minutes, plus 1 hour to chill

This slaw is a cool and refreshing salad that is sure to add a big crunch and vibrant color to your plate. Remember that fruits and vegetables provide a ton of fiber, vitamins, and minerals. The more color you include in your diet, the more nutrients you are providing to your body. Add a bit of spice to this dish by including some freshly ground black pepper or red pepper flakes.

3 cups shredded
green cabbage

2 cups shredded
red cabbage

2 cups jicama, cut in
¼-inch matchsticks

2 cups shredded carrots

½ cup chopped fresh
cilantro

¼ cup freshly squeezed
lemon or lime juice

2 tablespoons
extra-virgin olive oil

1 tablespoon honey

1. In a large bowl, combine the green cabbage, red cabbage, jicama, carrots, and cilantro.

2. In a small bowl or jar, combine the lemon juice, olive oil, and honey. Mix until well combined.

3. Pour the lemon mixture over the vegetables and toss to evenly coat the vegetables.

4. Cover the mixture and let sit in the refrigerator for about an hour for the flavors to combine and to soften the vegetables a bit. Serve chilled.

5. Store leftovers in an airtight container in the refrigerator for up to 3 days.

MAKE IT SIMPLER: Use a food processor with attachments to grate or shred the vegetables instead of chopping or shredding by hand.

PER SERVING (1 CUP): Calories: 67; Protein: 1g; Carbohydrates: 9g; Fiber: 2g; Total Fat: 4g; Saturated Fat: 1g; Sodium: 30mg; Cholesterol: 0mg; Potassium: 204mg; Phosphorus: 25mg

Crunchy Couscous Salad

DIABETES-FRIENDLY • HEART-HEALTHY • LOW-PROTEIN

SERVES 6 • **PREP TIME:** 15 minutes, plus optional
1 hour to chill • **COOK TIME:** 20 minutes

Couscous is a grain product made from durum wheat or semolina flour. It has a nutty and chewy texture. Couscous is extremely versatile and easy to prepare. Use it in salads like this recipe or serve it as a side dish with other proteins and vegetables. Substitute a can of low-sodium or no-salt-added chickpeas, red kidney beans, black beans, or tofu instead of using chicken for a vegetarian version.

1 cup couscous

6 ounces boneless, skinless chicken breast

6 cups water or low-sodium or no-salt-added chicken broth

1 medium cucumber, peeled with alternating green stripes, cut into slices and quartered

1 medium red bell pepper, diced

1 small yellow onion, diced

¼ cup chopped fresh parsley

¼ cup apple cider vinegar

3 tablespoons extra-virgin olive oil

1 teaspoon dried basil

½ teaspoon freshly ground black pepper

3 tablespoons crumbled feta cheese

1. Cook the couscous according to the package instructions.

2. Meanwhile, in a large pot over high heat, combine the chicken breast and water and bring to a boil. Cover the pot and reduce the heat to a gentle boil. Boil until the chicken breast is cooked through, about 15 minutes.

3. Remove the chicken from the pot, let cool, and then dice. In a large bowl, combine the couscous, chicken breast, cucumber, bell pepper, onion, and parsley and mix together.

4. In a separate bowl, combine the vinegar, oil, basil, and black pepper. Gently stir in the feta cheese. Mix the dressing with the couscous until combined. Enjoy warm or refrigerate for 1 hour and serve chilled.

5. Store leftovers in an airtight container in the refrigerator for up to 5 days.

PER SERVING (1 CUP): Calories: 149; Protein: 8.1g; Carbohydrates: 10g; Fiber: 2g; Total Fat: 9g; Saturated Fat: 2g; Sodium: 128mg; Cholesterol: 24mg; Potassium: 228mg; Phosphorus: 97mg

Tempeh Salad with Spicy Peanut Dressing

DIABETES-FRIENDLY • HEART-HEALTHY • MEDIUM-PROTEIN

SERVES 4 • **PREP TIME:** 20 minutes • **COOK TIME:** 10 minutes

Tempeh is a plant-based protein made from soybeans high in protein, prebiotics, vitamins, and minerals. If you don't like tempeh, use tofu, which has slightly less protein and potassium. Decrease the amount of maple syrup or brown rice noodles to lower the carbohydrate content if needed.

4 ounces brown rice noodles

2 cups fresh spinach

2 cups shredded red cabbage

2 medium carrots, grated

1 medium red bell pepper, thinly sliced

½ cup chopped fresh cilantro

¼ cup chopped fresh mint leaves

2 scallions, finely chopped

Avocado or olive oil cooking spray

4 ounces tempeh, cut into ½-inch strips

⅓ cup creamy unsalted peanut butter

¼ cup water

3 tablespoons coconut aminos

3 tablespoons maple syrup

Juice of 1 medium lime

1 small red chile, minced

1. Cook the brown rice noodles according to the package instructions, then rinse, drain, and transfer to a large mixing bowl.

2. Add the spinach, cabbage, carrots, bell pepper, cilantro, mint, and scallions to the bowl and toss together.

3. Spray a medium pan or skillet with cooking spray and heat over medium heat. Panfry the tempeh slices until they are browned on each side, about 3 minutes per side. Set aside.

4. In a small bowl, whisk together the peanut butter, water, coconut aminos, maple syrup, lime juice, and red chile. Mix until well combined and a dressing is formed.

5. Divide the rice noodle salad mixture and tempeh evenly among 4 plates. Top with the dressing and serve immediately.

PER SERVING (2 CUPS): Calories: 372; Protein: 13.7g; Carbohydrates: 55g; Fiber: 8g; Total Fat: 12g; Saturated Fat: 2g; Sodium: 371mg; Cholesterol: 0mg; Potassium: 536mg; Phosphorus: 47mg

Marinated Mustard Green Beans

DIABETES-FRIENDLY • HEART-HEALTHY • LOW-PROTEIN

SERVES 4 • PREP TIME: 5 minutes, plus 25 minutes to chill • **COOK TIME:** 5 minutes

Green beans are packed with fiber, vitamins, minerals, phytonutrients, and even some protein. The high-phytonutrient content of green beans means that they provide antioxidant and anti-inflammatory benefits. This recipe is designed to be eaten cold, but you can also warm it up if you prefer.

8½ cups water, divided

2 cups green beans, trimmed

½ cup red wine vinegar

2 teaspoons granulated sugar

½ teaspoon dry mustard

½ teaspoon dried oregano

½ teaspoon dried basil

¼ teaspoon freshly ground black pepper

¼ teaspoon salt

¼ cup finely chopped red onion

MAKE IT SIMPLER: You can use canned or frozen green beans and start at step 4. Look for the low-sodium, no-salt-added, not sauced or seasoned versions. If using canned beans, rinse them before using. If using frozen, thaw the beans or check the package instructions for how to prepare.

1. Prepare an ice bath in a large bowl.

2. In a large pot, bring 8 cups of water to a boil over high heat. Add the green beans and blanch for 3 to 5 minutes, until the beans are tender but still crisp.

3. Using a slotted spoon or strainer, transfer the green beans to the ice bath to cool. When cool, drain and pat dry.

4. In a small bowl or sauce jar, mix the vinegar, sugar, and mustard with ½ cup of water. Mix well until the mustard and sugar is dissolved.

5. Add the oregano, basil, pepper, and salt to the mustard mixture and stir until combined. Pour the mixture over the green beans and stir until well combined.

6. Sprinkle the red onion on top and let sit for 20 to 25 minutes in the refrigerator before serving.

7. Store leftovers in an airtight container in the refrigerator for up to 5 days.

PER SERVING (½ CUP): Calories: 45; Protein: 1.6g; Carbohydrates: 9g; Fiber: 2g; Total Fat: 1g; Saturated Fat: 0g; Sodium: 152mg; Cholesterol: 0mg; Potassium: 127mg; Phosphorus: 25mg

Cauliflower Mash

SERVES 6 • **PREP TIME:** 5 minutes • **COOK TIME:** 15 minutes

Mashed potatoes were something I loved to eat when growing up. Potatoes are still nice to enjoy from time to time, but they may add a bit too many carbohydrates and potassium into your diet. Cauliflower is a great alternative and provides a different nutrient profile. You can change up the flavor by using some of your favorite herbs/seasonings like Italian Seasoning Blend (page 136) or swap out the cream cheese for some plain yogurt.

1 medium head cauliflower, cut into florets

¼ cup low-fat cream cheese

¼ cup grated Parmesan cheese

2 garlic cloves, peeled

1 teaspoon extra-virgin olive oil

½ teaspoon freshly ground black pepper

1. Put a steamer basket in a large pot. Fill the pot with water to just below steamer basket. Bring water to a boil then add the cauliflower. Cover the pot and steam the cauliflower until tender, about 10 minutes.

2. Drain the cauliflower, transfer to a blender, and blend until smooth. Add the cream cheese, Parmesan cheese, garlic, oil, and pepper and blend again until well combined.

3. Remove from the blender and serve hot.

4. Store leftovers in an airtight container or resealable bag in the refrigerator for up to 3 days and in the freezer for up to 2 months.

MAKE IT SIMPLER: Instead of steaming the cauliflower on the stove, use a microwave. Put the cauliflower florets in a microwave-safe dish. Cover with a wet paper towel and cook on high until soft, about 8 to 10 minutes.

PER SERVING (½ CUP): Calories: 89; Protein: 4.2g; Carbohydrates: 7g; Fiber: 3g; Total Fat: 6g; Saturated Fat: 3g; Sodium: 124mg; Cholesterol: 13mg; Potassium: 203mg; Phosphorus: 78mg

Sesame Asparagus Spears

DIABETES-FRIENDLY • HEART-HEALTHY • LOW-PROTEIN

SERVES 4 • **PREP TIME:** 10 minutes • **COOK TIME:** 10 minutes

Asparagus is high in anti-inflammatory nutrients and antioxidants. Buy asparagus with rounded stalks, firm but thin stems, and closed tips. To trim the ends, try the bend-and-snap method: Hold up a spear horizontally and bend it with your hands gently. The spear will break at exactly where it should be trimmed.

1 tablespoon low-sodium soy sauce

1 tablespoon freshly squeezed lemon juice

2 garlic cloves, minced

1 teaspoon grated fresh ginger

1 teaspoon brown sugar

1 tablespoon olive or avocado oil

1 pound asparagus, trimmed and cut into 1½-inch pieces

1 teaspoon sesame oil

2 tablespoons sesame seeds

1 teaspoon freshly ground black pepper

½ teaspoon red pepper flakes (optional)

1. In a small bowl, whisk the soy sauce, lemon juice, garlic, ginger, and brown sugar until the brown sugar has dissolved.

2. In a large pan or skillet, heat the oil over medium-high heat. Add the asparagus and cook for about 3 minutes. Add the sauce mixture to the pan, stir together, and cook until the asparagus is tender but still crisp, about 4 minutes.

3. Remove the asparagus from the pan and divide among 4 plates. Drizzle the sesame oil over the asparagus and sprinkle the sesame seeds, black pepper, and red pepper flakes on top (if using). Serve immediately.

4. Store leftovers in an airtight container in the refrigerator for up to 4 days and in the freezer for up to 3 months.

MAKE IT LOWER IN POTASSIUM AND PHOSPHOROUS: Instead of using soy sauce, try coconut aminos. Coconut aminos is made from the fermented sap of coconut palm and has lower amounts of sodium, potassium, and phosphorus. It can be found in the same aisle as soy sauce.

PER SERVING (½ CUP): Calories: 107; Protein: 4.25g; Carbohydrates: 8g; Fiber: 3g; Total Fat: 8g; Saturated Fat: 1g; Sodium: 163mg; Cholesterol: 0mg; Potassium: 312mg; Phosphorus: 103mg

Roasted Napa Cabbage

DIABETES-FRIENDLY • HEART-HEALTHY • LOW-PROTEIN

SERVES 4 • **PREP TIME:** 5 minutes • **COOK TIME:** 15 minutes

Napa cabbage is a type of Chinese cabbage originating from China. It is commonly used in East Asian cuisine. This type of cabbage is oblong shaped with pale green leaves and a white stalk. Napa cabbage can be eaten raw or cooked, and it is commonly used for pickling or added to stir-fries or in soups. Napa has a mild taste raw but when cooked develops a sweeter flavor. Leave out the salt for a lower sodium content.

1 head Napa cabbage, quartered lengthwise

Avocado or olive oil cooking spray

2 tablespoons olive or avocado oil

2 tablespoons apple cider vinegar or lemon juice

2 tablespoons brown sugar

2 tablespoons Low-Sodium Dijon Mustard (page 139) or store-bought

1 teaspoon ground black pepper

¼ teaspoon salt

1 clove garlic, minced or grated

1. Preheat the oven to 450°. Line a baking sheet with parchment paper.

2. Spray the cabbage with cooking spray and put it, cut-side down, on the baking sheet.

3. Bake in the oven for 12 to 15 minutes, until the cabbage is wilted, warm, and slightly browned.

4. Meanwhile, in a small bowl, combine the olive oil, apple cider vinegar, brown sugar, mustard, pepper, salt, and garlic. Mix until well combined.

5. Remove the pan from the oven and brush the oil mixture onto the leaves.

6. Set the oven to broil. Return the pan to the oven and broil for 3 to 5 minutes, until browned and slightly caramelized. Serve whole or cut into smaller pieces.

7. Store leftovers in an airtight container in the refrigerator for up to 5 days.

PER SERVING (¼ OF CABBAGE): Calories: 173; Protein: 4.4g; Carbohydrates: 16g; Fiber 4g; Total Fat: 10g; Saturated Fat: 1g; Sodium: 171mg; Cholesterol: 0mg; Potassium: 600mg; Phosphorus: 122mg

Rice Pilaf

DIABETES-FRIENDLY • HEART-HEALTHY • LOW-PROTEIN
ONE POT • 5 INGREDIENTS OR FEWER

SERVES 4 • **PREP TIME:** 2 minutes • **COOK TIME:** 20 minutes

Rice pilaf is a side dish that can be paired with many meals. This recipe uses whole grains to make it more nutritious than traditional restaurant or boxed pilaf. You can even spice this up with more color and flavor by adding some of your favorite vegetables and seasonings to the pan when cooking or as a garnish on top.

2 teaspoons unsalted butter

¾ cup instant brown rice

¼ cup whole-wheat angel hair pasta, broken into ½-inch pieces

¼ cup instant wild rice

2 cups low-sodium or no-salt-added chicken or vegetable broth

1. In a large saucepan, melt the butter over medium heat. Add the brown rice, angel hair pasta, and wild rice.

2. Cook for about 3 minutes, stirring occasionally, until the ingredients are lightly toasted.

3. Add the chicken broth and bring to a boil. Reduce the heat to a simmer and cook for 10 to 12 minutes, until the rice and noodles are tender and the liquid is absorbed.

4. Remove the saucepan from the heat and let cool slightly. Fluff with a fork.

5. Store leftovers in an airtight container in the refrigerator for up to 4 days and in the freezer for up to 3 months.

MAKE IT SIMPLER: Instead of using both brown and wild rice, you can just use 1 cup of whichever rice you prefer or happen to have on hand.

PER SERVING (1 CUP): Calories: 113; Protein: 3.5g; Carbohydrates: 20g; Fiber: 1g; Total Fat: 3g; Saturated Fat: 1g; Sodium: 46mg; Cholesterol: 5mg; Potassium: 46mg; Phosphorus: 20mg

Vegan Sweet Potato Chili "Cheese" Fries

DIABETES-FRIENDLY • HEART-HEALTHY • MEDIUM-PROTEIN

SERVES 4 • PREP TIME: 10 minutes • **COOK TIME:** 45 minutes

This recipe is a healthier version of classic chili cheese fries. Sweet potatoes are a highly nutritious root vegetable that contain fiber, antioxidants, vitamins, and minerals, which help support immune function, as well as gut and brain health.

4 small sweet potatoes, cut into matchsticks

Avocado or olive oil cooking spray

1 medium orange bell pepper, roughly chopped

¾ cup plain Unsweetened Almond Milk (page 143) or store-bought

¼ cup raw cashews, soaked in hot water for 5 minutes, then drained

¼ cup chopped white onion

¼ cup no-salt-added or low-sodium canned cannellini beans

2 tablespoons nutritional yeast

1 tablespoon Taco Seasoning (page 134) or store-bought

1 (15-ounce) can low-sodium vegetarian bean chili

1. Preheat the oven to 425°F. Line a baking sheet with parchment paper and arrange the sweet potatoes in a single layer. Coat lightly with cooking spray.

2. Bake for 35 to 40 minutes, until crispy.

3. Meanwhile, in a blender, combine the bell pepper, almond milk, cashews, onion, beans, nutritional yeast, and taco seasoning. If you have a soup or hot setting on your blender, use that to make the sauce pureed and warm. If you don't have that setting, blend on high for 2 to 3 minutes until the mixture is smooth.

4. When the potatoes are ready, divide evenly among plates. Top each with chili and drizzle with the cheese sauce.

5. Store leftovers in the refrigerator for up to 3 days.

MAKE IT LOWER IN POTASSIUM: Put the cut potatoes in a large pot of warm water and let sit for 2 to 4 hours. Drain and pat dry before baking. This method is known as leaching, and research has shown that it can remove 50 to 75 percent of the potassium.

PER SERVING (½ CUP): Calories: 283; Protein: 12.6g; Carbohydrates: 41g; Fiber: 9g; Total Fat: 9g; Saturated Fat: 1g; Sodium: 210mg; Cholesterol: 0mg; Potassium: 571mg; Phosphorus: 112mg

Roasted Veggie Ginger Soup

DIABETES-FRIENDLY • HEART-HEALTHY • LOW-PROTEIN

SERVES 10 • **PREP TIME:** 10 minutes • **COOK TIME:** 50 minutes

This is a great soup for the cold fall and winter months. Try it with different toppings—add a dollop of plain Greek yogurt, whole-wheat croutons, a sprinkle of scallions, or grated Parmesan cheese.

3 cups spaghetti squash, peeled and cubed

6 medium carrots, peeled and quartered

1 garlic head, top cut off to expose the cloves inside

Avocado or olive oil cooking spray

2 tablespoons olive or avocado oil

1 medium yellow onion, diced

2 tablespoons grated fresh ginger

1 teaspoon ground cumin

½ teaspoon dried oregano

½ teaspoon dried thyme

Dash freshly ground black pepper

Dash salt

6 cups no-salt-added or low-sodium vegetable broth

1. Preheat the oven to 425°F. Line a baking sheet with parchment paper and arrange the spaghetti squash and carrots in a single layer. Wrap the garlic head in aluminum foil and set on the baking sheet. Spray the squash and carrots with a light coat of cooking spray and roast in the oven until cooked and lightly browned, 30 to 45 minutes.

2. When the vegetables are almost done, in a large pot, heat the oil over medium heat. Add the onions and ginger and cook for about 5 minutes until soft. Add the cumin, oregano, and thyme.

3. Remove the roasted vegetables and garlic from the oven. Squeeze the garlic cloves into the pot and add the roasted carrots and spaghetti squash. Mix together and season with pepper and salt.

4. Add the broth and bring the mixture to a boil. Once boiling, remove from the heat and puree using an immersion blender or placing in a regular blender. Serve immediately and enjoy.

5. Store leftovers in the refrigerator for up to 5 days. To freeze, cool the mixture and pour into a gallon-size resealable freezer bag. Lay it flat in the freezer for up to 3 months.

PER SERVING (1 CUP): Calories: 70; Protein: 0.8g; Carbohydrates: 11g; Fiber: 2g; Total Fat: 3g; Saturated Fat: 0.4g; Sodium: 167mg; Cholesterol: 0mg; Potassium: 211mg; Phosphorus: 23mg

Mushroom Soup

DIABETES-FRIENDLY • HEART-HEALTHY • LOW-PROTEIN • ONE POT

SERVES 4 • **PREP TIME:** 5 minutes • **COOK TIME:** 20 minutes

Traditional cream of mushroom soup is often high in sodium, saturated fat, and cholesterol. This recipe uses plant-based almond milk with flour and broth to create that creamy texture without the not-so-kidney-friendly ingredients. If you don't have vegan butter, use 3 tablespoons of unsalted butter plus 2 tablespoons of olive oil to keep the saturated fat content low.

5 tablespoons unsalted vegan butter

½ cup finely chopped white onion

1 cup thinly sliced or finely chopped white mushrooms

¼ cup whole-wheat flour

¼ cup all-purpose flour

2 cups no-salt-added or low-sodium chicken or vegetable broth

1 cup plain Unsweetened Almond Milk (page 143) or store-bought

½ teaspoon freshly ground black pepper

¼ teaspoon salt

1. In a medium pot, melt the butter over medium heat.

2. Add the onions and sauté for about 5 minutes, until soft and semi-translucent.

3. Add the mushrooms and cook for an additional 5 minutes until soft.

4. Sprinkle both flours over the mixture and stir for about 2 minutes.

5. Whisk in the broth and almond milk. Bring to a simmer and cook until thickened, about 5 minutes. Season with pepper and salt. Serve immediately and enjoy!

6. Store leftovers in the refrigerator for up to 5 days. To freeze, cool the mixture and pour into a gallon-size resealable freezer bag. Lay flat in the freezer for up to 3 months.

PER SERVING (¾ CUP): Calories: 274; Protein: 3.5g; Carbohydrates: 17g; Fiber: 3g; Total Fat: 22g; Saturated Fat: 10g; Sodium: 206mg; Cholesterol: 38mg; Potassium: 210mg; Phosphorus: 75mg

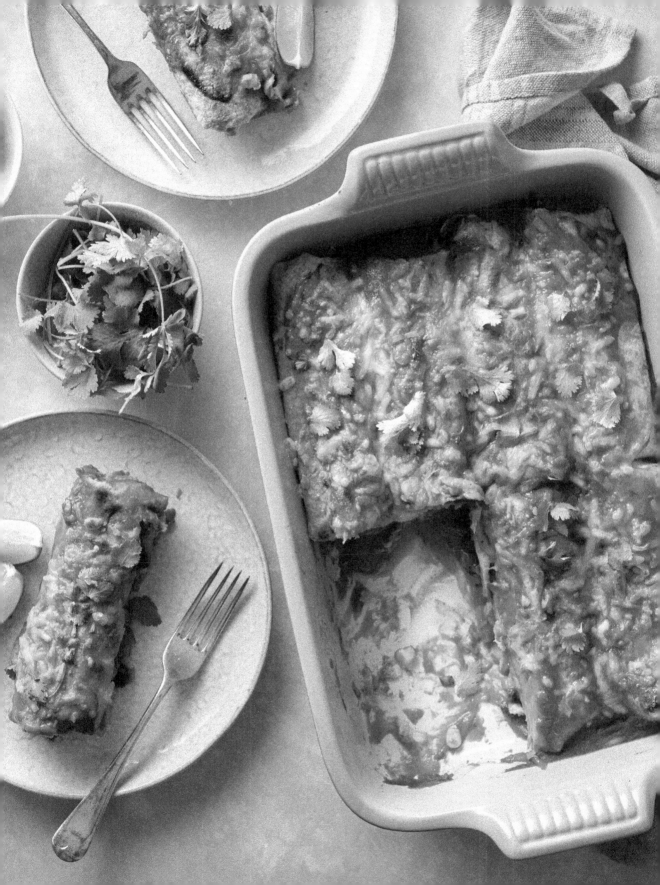

5

Vegetarian and Seafood Entrees

◀ Vegetarian Enchiladas, page 82

Slow Cooker Kabocha Barley Risotto

DIABETES-FRIENDLY • HEART-HEALTHY • LOW-PROTEIN

SERVES 6 • **PREP TIME:** 10 minutes • **COOK TIME:** 6 hours

Kabocha is a Japanese winter squash that is high in antioxidants and fiber, which is great for your gut health. It is a sweet squash that has a variety of uses in sweet and savory dishes. Although this is a winter squash, kabocha is available year-round and can be found at your local grocery store. When choosing your squash, pick one that feels heavier and has a deep green color.

2 teaspoons avocado or olive oil

½ small yellow onion, diced

2 garlic cloves, minced

Pinch freshly ground black pepper

8 ounces mushrooms, thinly sliced

1½ cups pearl barley, rinsed

3 cups kabocha squash, peeled, seeded, and cut into ¼-inch cubes

4 cups low-sodium or no-salt-added vegetable broth

1 cup frozen shelled edamame, thawed

1. In a medium skillet or pan, heat the oil over medium-high heat. Add the onion, garlic, and pepper. Stir occasionally and cook for about 5 minutes, until the onions are translucent.

2. Add the mushrooms and cook for about 2 minutes, until slightly brown and soft.

3. Add the barley and cook until the grain is slightly golden, about 2 minutes.

4. Transfer the ingredients to a 6-quart slow cooker. Add the squash and broth. Stir to combine.

5. Cover and cook over low heat for 5 to 6 hours, until the liquid is absorbed and the squash is fork-tender.

6. Stir in the edamame and serve immediately.

7. Store in an airtight container or resealable bag in the refrigerator for up to 5 days or in the freezer for up to 6 months. If storing in the freezer, I recommend using a resealable bag and lay it flat to freeze for easier storage.

MAKE IT SIMPLER: To make in a pressure cooker, set the pressure cooker to the sauté setting on high and add the oil, onion, garlic, and pepper. Cook until the onions are translucent, about 5 minutes. Add the mushrooms and stir occasionally. Cook for an additional 2 minutes, until the mushrooms are tender. Add the barley and cook for an additional minute, until the barley is slightly golden. Turn off the sauté setting and secure the lid. Set the pressure cooker to manual on high pressure and cook for 6 minutes. Let the pressure release naturally for 5 minutes and then quick release the remaining pressure.

PER SERVING (1½ CUPS): Calories: 212; Protein: 8.4g; Carbohydrates: 39g; Fiber: 9g; Total Fat: 3g; Saturated Fat: 1g; Sodium: 148mg; Cholesterol: 0mg; Potassium: 474mg; Phosphorus: 108mg

Chickpea Shawarma Wraps

DIABETES-FRIENDLY • HEART-HEALTHY • MEDIUM-PROTEIN

SERVES 4 • PREP TIME: 5 minutes • **COOK TIME:** 10 minutes

Though this looks like a long list of ingredients, this dish is actually very simple to make. Most of the ingredients are just seasonings and spices to give this dish a punch of flavor with no added salt. Chickpeas are a great plant-based protein source that are super versatile and affordable. You can enjoy this as is or swap out the pita for rice or naan bread.

FOR THE CHICKPEA SHAWARMA

1 (15-ounce) can no-salt-added or low-sodium chickpeas, drained, rinsed, and patted dry

½ teaspoon ground cumin

½ teaspoon salt

¼ teaspoon ground coriander

¼ teaspoon paprika

⅛ teaspoon ground cayenne pepper

⅛ teaspoon ground cinnamon

1 tablespoon olive or avocado oil

1 garlic clove, minced

Freshly ground black pepper

TO MAKE THE SHAWARMA

1. In a medium bowl, combine the chickpeas, cumin, salt, coriander, paprika, cayenne, and cinnamon. Mix together until chickpeas are well coated.

2. In a large skillet or pan, heat the oil over medium heat. Add the spiced chickpeas and the garlic. Cook, stirring occasionally, until warm and the chickpeas are crispy, about 10 minutes. Add black pepper to taste.

TO MAKE THE SAUCE

3. Meanwhile, in a small bowl, whisk the yogurt, cucumber, lemon juice, garlic, and cumin.

FOR THE SAUCE

1 cup plain nonfat Greek yogurt

½ cup cucumber, seeded, peeled, and finely chopped

1 tablespoon freshly squeezed lemon juice

1 garlic clove, minced

1 teaspoon ground cumin

FOR THE WRAPS

4 medium (6-inch) whole-wheat pita pockets

8 leaves romaine lettuce

1 small tomato, cut into 8 thin rounds

¼ medium red onion, thinly sliced (optional)

TO MAKE THE WRAPS

4. Toast the pitas in a toaster oven, then assemble the pita pockets. To each pita pocket, add 2 leaves of lettuce, 2 slices of tomato, one-quarter of the chickpea mixture, and drizzle with some sauce. Top with red onion (if using).

5. Store leftovers of the chickpea mixture in the refrigerator for up to 5 days or in the freezer for up to 3 months.

PER SERVING (1 WRAP): Calories: 216; Protein: 13.4g; Carbohydrates: 29g; Fiber: 6g; Total Fat: 6g; Saturated Fat: 1g; Sodium: 384mg; Cholesterol: 3mg; Potassium: 352mg; Phosphorus: 141mg

Roasted Vegetable and Tofu Fried Rice

DIABETES-FRIENDLY • HEART-HEALTHY • MEDIUM-PROTEIN

SERVES 6 • **PREP TIME:** 15 minutes • **COOK TIME:** 45 minutes

Fried rice is a super easy dish to make that incorporates vegetables, grains, and protein. You can easily customize it by swapping in your favorite vegetables or using whatever you have on hand. I like to make fried rice at the end of the week when I'm trying to use up my weekly groceries. Just chop up some veggies, roast them, and quickly sauté together with some protein and rice. Purchase coconut aminos with no added sodium.

1 medium eggplant, cubed

1 medium zucchini, diced

1 medium red bell pepper, sliced

1 medium unpeeled sweet potato, diced

14 ounces firm tofu, diced

Avocado or olive oil cooking spray

2 tablespoons coconut aminos

1 tablespoon rice vinegar

1 tablespoon light brown sugar

1 tablespoon minced fresh ginger

1 tablespoon sesame oil

2 garlic cloves, minced

1. Preheat the oven to 400°F and line 2 baking sheets with parchment paper.

2. Arrange the eggplant, zucchini, bell pepper, and sweet potato in a single layer on one baking sheet and the tofu in a single layer on the other baking sheet. Spray with oil on top of everything. Toss to coat.

3. Place both sheets in the oven and bake for about 30 minutes, until the vegetables are roasted and the tofu is crispy and golden brown around the edges.

4. In a small bowl, whisk the coconut aminos, rice vinegar, brown sugar, and ginger.

5. In a large wok or skillet, heat the sesame oil over medium heat. Add the garlic and sauté for 30 to 45 seconds until fragrant.

6. Add the eggs and scramble until cooked through, about 5 minutes. If using packaged rice, heat it up in the microwave to the desired temperature.

2 large eggs, beaten

**2 cups cooked
brown rice**

**2 cups cauliflower
rice, thawed**

7. Stir in the cooked brown rice and cauliflower rice, and cook, stirring frequently, for 2 minutes.

8. Add the roasted vegetables and drizzle the coconut amino sauce on top. Gently mix together and cook for an additional 3 minutes.

9. Remove from the heat and divide into 6 servings. Add the tofu on top and serve immediately.

10. Leftovers can be kept in an airtight container in the refrigerator for up to 3 days and in the freezer for up to 3 months.

PER SERVING (1½ CUPS): Calories: 276; Protein: 11.5g; Carbohydrates: 36g; Fiber: 5g; Total Fat: 10g; Saturated Fat: 2g; Sodium: 149mg; Cholesterol: 62mg; Potassium: 453mg; Phosphorus: 131mg

Vegetarian Garam Masala Burritos

DIABETES-FRIENDLY • HEART-HEALTHY • LOW-PROTEIN

SERVES 6 • **PREP TIME:** 15 minutes • **COOK TIME:** 30 minutes

Garam masala is a blend of fragrant and flavorful ground spices from India. It is commonly used in Indian, Pakistani, Nepalese, and Sri Lankan cuisines. It contains a wide variety of fragrant flavorful spices. You can find it at most local grocery stores or online.

1 tablespoon olive or avocado oil

2 cups yellow potatoes, cubed

1 cup low-sodium or no-salt-added vegetable broth

1 medium tomato, diced

2 garlic cloves, minced

2 teaspoons minced fresh ginger

1 teaspoon ground cumin

½ teaspoon ground coriander

½ teaspoon ground turmeric

14 ounces firm tofu, drained and patted dry

1 cup plain frozen mixed vegetables

¼ cup chopped fresh cilantro

½ teaspoon garam masala

6 (10-inch) whole-grain tortillas

1. In a large skillet, heat the oil over medium heat. Add the potatoes and cook until lightly browned, about 1 minute.

2. Add the vegetable broth and cover to let the potatoes cook until tender, about 15 minutes. Stir occasionally.

3. Add the tomato, garlic, ginger, cumin, coriander, and turmeric. Cook for 2 to 3 minutes. Crumble in the tofu and cook for an additional 4 minutes.

4. Add the mixed vegetables, cilantro, and garam masala. Stir gently and cook until the vegetables and mixture are all warm, about 3 minutes. Remove from the heat and let cool slightly.

5. Assemble the burritos: Spoon about ⅓ cup of the filling onto the middle of the tortilla. Roll the burrito by tucking in the ends and rolling up to wrap tightly. Repeat for all the burritos.

6. Leftover burritos can be wrapped in foil and kept in the refrigerator for up to 5 days and in freezer in an airtight resealable bag for up to 6 months.

PER SERVING (1 BURRITO): Calories: 295; Protein: 10.5g; Carbohydrates: 43g; Fiber: 4g; Total Fat: 10g; Saturated Fat: 1g; Sodium: 253mg; Cholesterol: 0mg; Potassium: 638mg; Phosphorus: 69mg

"Cheezy" Pasta with Broccoli

DIABETES-FRIENDLY • HEART-HEALTHY • MEDIUM-PROTEIN

SERVES 4 • **PREP TIME:** 10 minutes • **COOK TIME:** 30 minutes

This pasta mimics macaroni and cheese. Instead of traditional cheese, however, this recipe uses nutritional yeast, which has a cheesy, nutty flavor and is a complete protein. Nutritional yeast is sold as flakes, granules, or powder, and is usually found in the spice section. If you need to reduce the carbohydrate content, decrease the portion of pasta and substitute with your favorite kidney-friendly vegetable.

12 ounces whole-wheat pasta

1 tablespoon avocado oil

2 garlic cloves, minced

1 small carrot, peeled and diced

½ cup minced white onion

1 (15-ounce) can no-salt-added or low-sodium white beans, drained and rinsed

1 cup low-sodium or no-salt-added vegetable broth, plus more as needed

2 rounded tablespoons nutritional yeast

1 tablespoon white vinegar or lemon juice

½ teaspoon salt

½ teaspoon freshly ground black pepper

4 cups broccoli florets

1. Bring a large pot of water to a boil and cook the pasta according to the package instructions.

2. Meanwhile, in a large pan, heat the oil and garlic over medium heat. Add the carrot and onion and cook for about 5 minutes, until soft. Remove from the heat and pour into a food processor or blender.

3. Add the beans, broth, nutritional yeast, vinegar, salt, and pepper to the blender. Puree until creamy and smooth with a sauce-like texture. Set aside.

4. When there is about 3 minutes left on the pasta, add the broccoli to the pot.

5. Drain the water out of the pot and add the sauce to the pasta and broccoli. Stir to combine. You can add more vegetable broth or reserve some pasta water to thin out the sauce if needed. Serve.

6. Store leftovers in an airtight container in the refrigerator for up to 5 days.

PER SERVING (2 CUPS): Calories: 307; Protein: 14.9g; Carbohydrates: 52g; Fiber: 13g; Total Fat: 7g; Saturated Fat: 1g; Sodium: 281mg; Cholesterol: 0mg; Potassium: 683mg; Phosphorus: 277mg

Tangy Kale Orzo with Tempeh Sausage

DIABETES-FRIENDLY • HEART-HEALTHY • MEDIUM-PROTEIN

SERVES 4 • **PREP TIME:** 5 minutes • **COOK TIME:** 15 minutes

Orzo is a rice-shaped pasta made from wheat semolina flour and is often used in soups or rice pilaf. I love the chewy and tender texture of orzo. If you don't have time to make your own salt-free Italian Seasoning Blend (page 136), Walmart's brand Great Value has an Italian seasoning blend that is also sodium-free. Omit the salt in this recipe if desired.

16 ounces whole-wheat orzo pasta

1 tablespoon avocado or olive oil

8 ounces tempeh, crumbled

2 garlic cloves, minced

½ teaspoon dried parsley

½ teaspoon Italian Seasoning Blend (page 136) or store-bought

½ teaspoon onion powder

¼ teaspoon smoked paprika

3 cups roughly chopped fresh kale

Juice of 3 medium lemons

¼ teaspoon salt

¼ teaspoon freshly ground black pepper

1. Bring a medium pot of water to a boil and cook the orzo pasta according to the package instructions.

2. Meanwhile, in a large pan or skillet, heat the oil over medium heat. Add the tempeh and garlic. Add the parsley, Italian seasoning, onion powder, and paprika and stir to coat the tempeh. Gently cook for 5 to 6 minutes until browned.

3. Add the kale and sauté until the kale is wilted, about 2 minutes. Squeeze lemon juice over the pan.

4. When the orzo is done cooking, drain the water and return to the pot. Add the tempeh and kale to the orzo and toss to combine. Season with salt and pepper and serve immediately.

5. Store leftovers in an airtight container in the refrigerator for up to 5 days and in the freezer for up to 6 months.

PER SERVING (1½ CUPS): Calories: 314; Protein: 18.6g; Carbohydrates: 46g; Fiber: 11g; Total Fat: 9g; Saturated Fat: 1g; Sodium: 164mg; Cholesterol: 0mg; Potassium: 387mg; Phosphorus: 163mg

Spicy Black Bean Power Bowls

DIABETES-FRIENDLY • HEART-HEALTHY • MEDIUM-PROTEIN

SERVES 4 • **PREP TIME:** 5 minutes • **COOK TIME:** 15 minutes

This black bean power bowl is super easy to put together and packed with fiber and nutrients. Spice it up with red pepper flakes or Siete brand hot sauce and a dollop of plain yogurt. Or make your own pico de gallo instead of using store-bought for a lower-sodium option: Dice 2 Roma tomatoes and mince one-quarter of a small red onion, 1 jalapeño pepper (optional), 1 garlic clove, and 1 tablespoon of fresh cilantro. Mix together with 1 to 2 tablespoons of fresh lime juice and add pepper to taste.

1 cup fresh pico de gallo

1 (15-ounce) can no-salt-added or low-sodium black beans, drained and rinsed

½ teaspoon ground cumin

½ teaspoon ground cayenne pepper or chili powder

1 tablespoon olive oil or avocado oil

2 garlic cloves, minced

4 cups finely chopped mustard greens

2 cups cooked brown rice

½ cup low-sodium salsa

4 tablespoons crumbled feta cheese

1. In a large pan or skillet over medium heat, sauté the pico de gallo for 2 to 3 minutes, until soft.

2. Add the black beans, cumin, and cayenne and stir together, gently mashing some of the beans. Cook until warm and slightly thickened, about 5 minutes. Remove from the skillet and set aside.

3. In the same pan, heat the oil and garlic over medium heat. Cook for about 45 seconds, until the garlic is fragrant. Add the mustard greens and cook for 4 to 5 minutes, until tender. If using premade or packaged rice, heat it up in the microwave to the desired temperature.

4. Assemble the bowls: Put ½ cup of cooked brown rice, one-quarter of the mustard greens, one-quarter of the black beans and top each bowl with 2 tablespoons of salsa and 1 tablespoon of feta cheese.

5. Store leftovers in an airtight container in the refrigerator for up to 5 days or in the freezer for up to 3 months.

PER SERVING (1 BOWL): Calories: 319; Protein: 12.7g; Carbohydrates: 54g; Fiber: 11g; Total Fat: 7g; Saturated Fat: 2g; Sodium: 218mg; Cholesterol: 8mg; Potassium: 609mg; Phosphorus: 184mg

Vegetarian Enchiladas

DIABETES-FRIENDLY • HEART-HEALTHY • MEDIUM-PROTEIN

SERVES 8 • PREP TIME: 5 minutes • **COOK TIME:** 35 minutes

This vegetarian dish is filling and jam-packed with veggies. The nutrition content may vary depending on how much enchilada sauce you actually consume. You can use store-bought if you don't have time to make your own sauce, but choose a low-sodium product with minimal ingredients. Serve garnished with lime wedges, if desired.

Avocado or olive oil cooking spray

2 tablespoons avocado or olive oil

2 cups diced zucchini

1 (10-ounce) package frozen corn

1 small red onion, diced

1 (15-ounce) can no-salt-added or low-sodium black beans, drained and rinsed

3 cups Enchilada Sauce (page 142) or store-bought, divided

8 (10-inch) whole-wheat tortillas

2 cups shredded low-sodium mozzarella or Mexican-blend cheese

Handful chopped cilantro, for garnish (optional)

1. Preheat the oven to 350°F. Coat a 13-by-9-inch baking dish with cooking spray and set aside.

2. In a large skillet or pan, heat the oil over medium-high heat. Add the zucchini, corn, and onion and sauté until the vegetables are soft, about 5 minutes. Add the beans, stir gently, and cook for an additional 1 to 2 minutes. Remove from the heat.

3. Spread about 1 cup of the enchilada sauce on the bottom of the baking dish. Take 1 tortilla and spread about ½ cup of the bean mixture onto the center of the tortilla. Sprinkle about 2 tablespoons of cheese and roll up the tortilla. Place the tortilla seam-side down in the baking dish. Repeat with all of the tortillas.

4. Sprinkle with the remaining ¼ cup cheese and top with the remaining enchilada sauce. Cover with foil and bake for 20 minutes. Uncover and bake for an additional 10 minutes. Garnish with cilantro (if using) and serve.

5. Store leftovers in an airtight container in the refrigerator for up to 5 days or in the freezer for up to 3 months.

PER SERVING (1 ENCHILADA): Calories: 316; Protein: 15.3g; Carbohydrates: 39g; Fiber: 9g; Total Fat: 13g; Saturated Fat: 5g; Sodium: 318mg; Cholesterol: 18mg; Potassium: 453mg; Phosphorus: 204mg

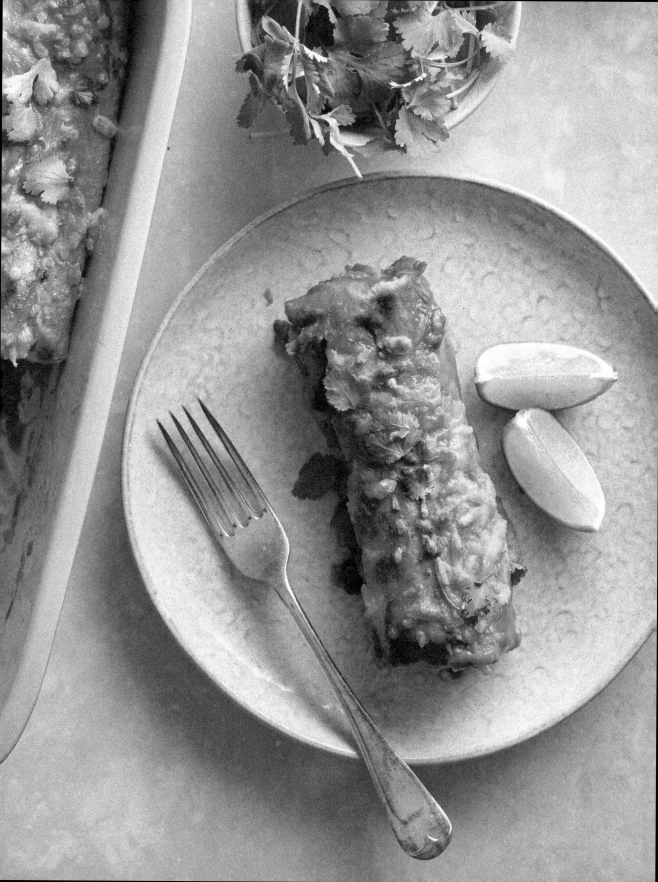

Pressure Cooker Lentil Sloppy Joes with Coleslaw

DIABETES-FRIENDLY • HEART-HEALTHY • MEDIUM-PROTEIN

SERVES 6 • **PREP TIME:** 10 minutes • **COOK TIME:** 45 minutes

This recipe is a healthy twist on a classic American favorite. Though the list of ingredients looks long, this dish is actually very easy to make. If you need to decrease the carbohydrate content, try making an open-faced sandwich instead by using only half of the bun. If you don't have a pressure cooker, you can use a slow cooker. Simply add all the ingredients to the pot, cover, and cook on high for 3½ hours. If cooking on the stovetop, sauté the vegetables in a stockpot over medium heat, add the remaining ingredients, and mix well. Cover with a lid and let simmer for 1 hour.

FOR THE SLOPPY JOES

1 teaspoon avocado oil

1 medium onion, diced

1 medium red bell pepper, diced

2 garlic cloves, minced

2 cups low-sodium or no-salt-added vegetable broth

1 (15-ounce) can low-sodium or no-salt-added diced tomatoes

1 cup dry lentils (green or brown), rinsed

2 tablespoons low-sodium or no-salt-added tomato paste

1 tablespoon maple syrup

TO MAKE THE SLOPPY JOES

1. On the pressure cooker, select the sauté setting on high. Sauté the oil, onion, bell pepper, and garlic for 3 minutes, until the vegetables are soft.

2. Add the broth, tomatoes and their juices, lentils, tomato paste, maple syrup, mustard, paprika, chili powder, cumin, lemon juice, and coconut aminos. Stir and mix well. Close the lid and pressure cook on high for 15 minutes.

TO MAKE THE COLESLAW

3. Meanwhile, in a medium bowl, whisk the mustard, vinegar, and black pepper. Add the coleslaw and toss gently.

4. Let the pressure release naturally for 15 minutes. Manually release any remaining pressure.

1 tablespoon Low-Sodium
Dijon Mustard (page 139)
or store-bought

1 teaspoon
smoked paprika

1 teaspoon chili powder

1 teaspoon ground cumin

1 teaspoon freshly
squeezed lemon juice

1 teaspoon
coconut aminos

6 whole-wheat
hamburger buns

FOR THE COLESLAW

2 tablespoons
Low-Sodium Dijon
Mustard (page 139) or
store-bought

2 tablespoons apple
cider vinegar

¼ teaspoon freshly
ground black pepper

4 cups bagged
coleslaw mix

5. Portion out the lentil mixture onto the buns. You can either top the sloppy joes with coleslaw or serve it on the side.

6. Store the leftover lentil mixture in an airtight container in the refrigerator for up to 1 week or in the freezer for up to 3 months.

MAKE IT LOWER IN POTASSIUM: Soak the dry lentils in a bowl of water overnight. Discard the liquid then continue with the recipe. Soaking the lentils overnight will leach out some of the potassium.

PER SERVING (1 SANDWICH + ⅔ CUP COLESLAW): Calories: 320; Protein: 15.5g; Carbohydrates: 51g; Fiber: 11g; Total Fat: 5g; Saturated Fat: 1g; Sodium: 268mg; Cholesterol: 0mg; Potassium: 814mg; Phosphorus: 295mg

Tofu Spring Rolls

DIABETES-FRIENDLY • HEART-HEALTHY • MEDIUM-PROTEIN

SERVES 3 • **PREP TIME:** 10 minutes • **COOK TIME:** 15 minutes

Spring rolls are super easy to make, and can be customized to your liking. Try using any of your favorite kidney-friendly vegetables and other proteins, or use raw tofu instead of frying. If you'd like a dipping sauce for these spring rolls, two tablespoons per serving of Peanut Apple Sauce (page 141) would be tasty. Different brands of tofu and rice paper will contain different ingredients which will affect the nutrition content. Be sure to choose a product that is low in sodium, potassium, and has the appropriate carbohydrate content to fit your needs.

6 cups water

14 ounces firm tofu, drained and patted dry

½ tablespoon ground cumin

½ tablespoon garlic powder

½ teaspoon freshly ground black pepper

¼ teaspoon salt

1 tablespoon olive or avocado oil

12 rice paper wrappers

12 leaves romaine lettuce, washed, and each leaf halved lengthwise

2 medium carrots, peeled and thinly sliced

2 medium red bell peppers, thinly sliced

1 medium cucumbers, thinly sliced

1. In a medium pot, boil the water and set aside to cool slightly. You will be using this water to soak the rice papers later.

2. Cut the tofu into 12 even pieces lengthwise and spread evenly on a plate.

3. In a small bowl, mix together the cumin, garlic powder, black pepper, and salt. Season the tofu evenly on both sides with the spice mixture.

4. In a medium pan or skillet, heat the oil over medium heat. Put the tofu strips in a single layer on the pan. Fry each side until lightly browned, 1 to 2 minutes on each side. Remove the tofu from the pan and set aside to cool.

5. Pour the slightly cooled water into a shallow pan. Immerse a piece of rice paper in the water for about 5 seconds. The paper may still be a bit hard, but it will continue to soften as you prepare the dish.

6. Transfer the wet rice paper to a damp towel or damp cutting board. Add 2 halves of lettuce in the center of the wrapper. Add some carrots, bell peppers, and cucumbers on top of the lettuce. Set 1 cooled tofu strip on top of the vegetables.

7. Fold the sides of the rice paper in and then roll from the bottom up. Make sure the roll is tight. Repeat with the remaining pieces of rice paper.

8. Serve immediately and enjoy.

MAKE IT SIMPLER: Try eating some rolls deconstructed without the paper, or use iceberg or romaine lettuce as your wrap instead.

PER SERVING (4 SPRING ROLLS): Calories: 322; Protein: 18g; Carbohydrates: 41g; Fiber: 8g; Total Fat: 11g; Saturated Fat: 2g; Sodium: 324mg; Cholesterol: 0mg; Potassium: 446mg; Phosphorus: 64mg

Feta, Onion, and Pepper Pizza

DIABETES-FRIENDLY • HEART-HEALTHY • MEDIUM-PROTEIN • ONE POT

SERVES 4 • PREP TIME: 10 minutes • **COOK TIME:** 15 minutes

Pizza is one of my favorite foods and I love that it can be a part of a healthy renal diet. Make your own at home so that you are in control and able to customize it to make sure you stay within your nutrient goals. If you don't have time to make your own pizza dough, you can purchase a low-sodium premade dough (make sure it has simple ingredients), or use whole-wheat tortillas or a whole-grain flatbread. If using the tortillas or flatbread, lower the temp to 350°F and cook for the same amount of time. Substitute low-sodium mozzarella cheese for the feta cheese to lower the fat and sodium content if needed.

1 recipe Salt-Free Pizza Dough (page 144) or store-bought

2 tablespoons avocado oil

3 medium red bell peppers, diced

1 cup sliced red onion

2 garlic cloves, minced

½ cup crumbled feta cheese

1 teaspoon Italian Seasoning Blend (page 136) or store-bought

½ cup fresh basil leaves, for garnish (optional)

1. Preheat the oven to 450°F. Put the pizza crust on a pizza pan or baking sheet.

2. Spread the oil over the crust and arrange the bell peppers, onions, and garlic on top. Sprinkle with the feta and Italian seasoning.

3. Bake for 10 to 12 minutes, until the vegetables are crispy and tender.

4. Let cool for 2 to 3 minutes, cut into 12 slices, garnish with basil leaves (if using), and enjoy.

5. Store leftovers in the refrigerator in an airtight container for up to 5 days.

PER SERVING (3 SLICES): Calories: 425; Protein: 11.1g; Carbohydrates: 62g; Fiber: 4g; Total Fat: 15g; Saturated Fat: 4g; Sodium: 224mg; Cholesterol: 17mg; Potassium: 301mg; Phosphorus: 174mg

Shrimp Quesadillas

DIABETES-FRIENDLY • MEDIUM-PROTEIN

SERVES 2 • **PREP TIME:** 10 minutes, plus 15 minutes to marinate • **COOK TIME:** 10 minutes

Shrimp can be a good source of protein to include in your renal diet. Fresh or frozen is always best. You can also customize this recipe and swap out the shrimp for one of your favorite proteins like fish or beans.

5 ounces raw shrimp, peeled and deveined

2 tablespoons chopped fresh cilantro, plus more for garnish

1 tablespoon freshly squeezed lime juice

¼ teaspoon ground cumin

⅛ teaspoon ground cayenne pepper

2 tablespoons plain nonfat Greek yogurt

2 (10-inch) flour tortillas

2 tablespoons shredded low-sodium mozzarella or Mexican-blend cheese

Lime wedges, for garnish (optional)

1. Rinse the shrimp and cut into bite-size pieces.

2. In a small bowl or resealable bag, combine the cilantro, lime juice, cumin, and cayenne. Add the shrimp and mix well. Let the shrimp marinate for 15 minutes.

3. In a medium sauté pan, heat the shrimp over medium heat. Cook and stir frequently for 2 minutes, or until the shrimp turns orange. Remove from the heat and mix in the yogurt.

4. In a large pan, heat 1 tortilla on both sides over low-medium heat. Add half of the shrimp mixture and sprinkle with 1 tablespoon of cheese.

5. Fold the tortilla in half and turn over in the skillet to cook for 2 minutes. Remove from the pan. Repeat steps 4 and 5 for the second quesadilla.

6. Cut each quesadilla into 4 pieces. Garnish with the extra cilantro and lime wedges (optional) before serving.

MAKE IT LOWER IN PROTEIN: Decrease the amount of shrimp you use in the recipe. You can substitute it with some kidney-friendly vegetables to add some bulk to the meal. Try carrots or cauliflower and marinate in the sauce just like the shrimp.

PER SERVING (1 QUESADILLA): Calories: 221; Protein: 17.7g; Carbohydrates: 25g; Fiber: 0g; Total Fat: 6g; Saturated Fat: 1g; Sodium: 285mg; Cholesterol: 96mg; Potassium: 205mg; Phosphorus: 183mg

Baked Crab Cakes with Corn and Roasted Broccoli

DIABETES-FRIENDLY • HEART-HEALTHY • HIGH-PROTEIN

SERVES 4 • PREP TIME: 10 minutes • **COOK TIME:** 20 minutes

Crab cakes are fun and remind me of a beach vacation. This crab cake recipe is lightened up with vegetables and baked instead of fried. Compared to restaurant versions, this one is much lower in sodium and contains more fiber. You can easily customize this recipe with any of your favorite vegetables and seasonings.

1 large egg

1 large egg white or 2 tablespoons liquid egg whites

¼ cup plain nonfat Greek yogurt

Juice of 1 medium lemon

1 tablespoon Low-Sodium Dijon Mustard (page 139) or store-bought

½ teaspoon paprika

¼ teaspoon freshly ground black pepper

8 ounces crabmeat

½ cup finely chopped celery

½ cup finely chopped sweet onion

½ cup finely chopped red bell pepper

2 garlic cloves, minced

¾ cup whole-wheat panko bread crumbs

1. Preheat the oven to 400°F and line 2 baking sheets with parchment paper.

2. In a large bowl, mix the egg, egg white, yogurt, lemon juice, mustard, paprika, and black pepper. Stir in the crabmeat, celery, onion, bell pepper, and garlic.

3. Gently stir in the bread crumbs until just combined. Using your hands, form the mixture into 10 patties and put on one of the prepared baking sheets.

4. Lightly brush the top of each crab cake with oil and set aside.

5. Put the broccoli onto the other prepared baking sheet. Spray with cooking spray and sprinkle with the seasoning. Gently toss to coat and place both baking sheets in oven.

6. Bake for 15 to 20 minutes, until the crab cakes are golden brown on top and the broccoli is slightly browned and cooked through.

2 teaspoons avocado or
olive oil

2½ cups broccoli florets

Avocado or olive oil cooking spray

1 tablespoon Trader Joe's
21 Seasoning Salute or
no-sodium seasoning
of choice

4 medium corn cobs,
husks and silks removed

Lemon wedges,
for garnish

Siete brand hot sauce,
for dipping

7. Meanwhile, fill a large stockpot a little over halfway with water and place it over high heat. Bring to a boil and add the corn on the cob. Cover and cook for 5 to 7 minutes until done.

8. Serve 2 crab cakes with ½ cup of broccoli and 1 corn cob. Garnish with some lemon wedges and hot sauce.

9. Store leftovers in an airtight container in the refrigerator for up to 5 days or in the freezer for up to 3 months.

MAKE IT SIMPLER: Use a food processor to chop your vegetables to cut down on prep time and manual labor.

PER SERVING (2 CRAB CAKES + ½ CUP BROCCOLI + 1 CORN):
Calories: 309; Protein: 20.7g; Carbohydrates: 44g; Fiber: 8g;
Total Fat: 8g; Saturated Fat: 1g; Sodium: 166mg; Cholesterol: 101mg;
Potassium: 698 mg; Phosphorus: 216mg

Zesty Tuna Salad Sandwiches with Carrot Sticks

DIABETES-FRIENDLY • HEART-HEALTHY • HIGH-PROTEIN • ONE POT

SERVES 4 • PREP TIME: 15 minutes

This recipe uses more veggies and yogurt for added nutrients, probiotics, and fiber than a classic tuna salad. I like to use the brand Wild Planet for my tuna because they harvest sustainably and are environmentally conscious. Their products are also higher in nutritional value. You can find Wild Planet tuna at most local grocery stores.

1 (5-ounce) can no-salt-added albacore tuna, drained and rinsed

½ cup plain nonfat yogurt

¼ cup chopped fresh parsley or cilantro

1 celery stalk, diced

1 mini cucumber, diced

1 small radish, diced

1 scallions, green part only, diced

Juice of ½ lemon

¼ teaspoon freshly ground black pepper

4 tablespoons Low-Sodium Dijon Mustard (page 139) or store-bought (optional)

8 Ezekiel 4:9 low-sodium sprouted whole-grain bread slices

4 ounces carrot sticks

1. In a large mixing bowl, combine the tuna, yogurt, parsley, celery, cucumber, radish, scallion, lemon juice, and pepper. Mix together until well combined.

2. Toast the bread to your desired doneness and spread on 1 tablespoon of mustard onto one slice of toast. Evenly divide the tuna salad among 4 slices of toast and set the other slices of toast on top.

3. Serve each sandwich with 1 ounce of carrot sticks.

MAKE IT SIMPLER: Use a food processer to quickly and easily chop up all the veggies and herbs.

MAKE IT LOWER IN PROTEIN: Lower the protein content in this recipe by using less tuna or making an open-faced sandwich with just one slice of toast. Using only one slice of toast will also lower the potassium content of this recipe.

PER SERVING (1 SANDWICH): Calories: 320; Protein: 19.4g; Carbohydrates: 34g; Fiber: 8g; Total Fat: 14g; Saturated Fat: 2g; Sodium: 201mg; Cholesterol: 23mg; Potassium: 408mg; Phosphorus: 153mg

Sheet Pan Teriyaki Salmon with Roasted Vegetables

DIABETES-FRIENDLY • HEART-HEALTHY • MEDIUM-PROTEIN • ONE POT

SERVES 2 • **PREP TIME:** 10 minutes, plus 2 hours to marinate • **COOK TIME:** 30 minutes

Salmon is a great source of healthy fats, vitamin B_{12}, and protein. The omega-3 fats in salmon are good for lowering inflammation and blood pressure. Wild-caught salmon contains more nutrients and fewer contaminants than farmed. Garnish with chopped parsley or cilantro, if desired.

4 ounces wild-caught salmon fillets

½ cup Mango Teriyaki Sauce (page 140)

2 cups eggplant, cut into 1-inch pieces

1 medium carrot, cut into ½-inch pieces

1 medium turnip, cut into ½-inch pieces

2 tablespoons sesame oil

½ teaspoon ground ginger

½ teaspoon garlic powder

1. Put the salmon fillets in a gallon-size resealable bag and marinate in the mango teriyaki sauce for 2 hours.

2. Preheat the oven to 400°F. Line a baking sheet with parchment paper and spread out the eggplant, carrot, and turnip on it. Drizzle with sesame oil and season with the ginger and garlic powder. Toss until everything is well coated.

3. Roast for 15 to 20 minutes until slightly tender. Remove from the oven and flip the vegetables over. Add the marinated salmon to the same sheet and bake for an additional 10 minutes, until everything is cooked through.

4. Store leftovers in an airtight container in the refrigerator for up to 5 days or in the freezer for up to 3 months.

MAKE IT LOWER IN PROTEIN, POTASSIUM, AND PHOSPHORUS: Decrease the size of the salmon filet by 1 or 2 ounces depending on your needs. Add more veggies, like colorful bell peppers or sugar snap peas, or use a plant-based protein instead.

PER SERVING (½ OF RECIPE): Calories: 373; Protein: 19.7g; Carbohydrates: 25g; Fiber: 5g; Total Fat: 23g; Saturated Fat: 3g; Sodium: 156mg; Cholesterol: 50mg; Potassium: 815mg; Phosphorus: 230mg

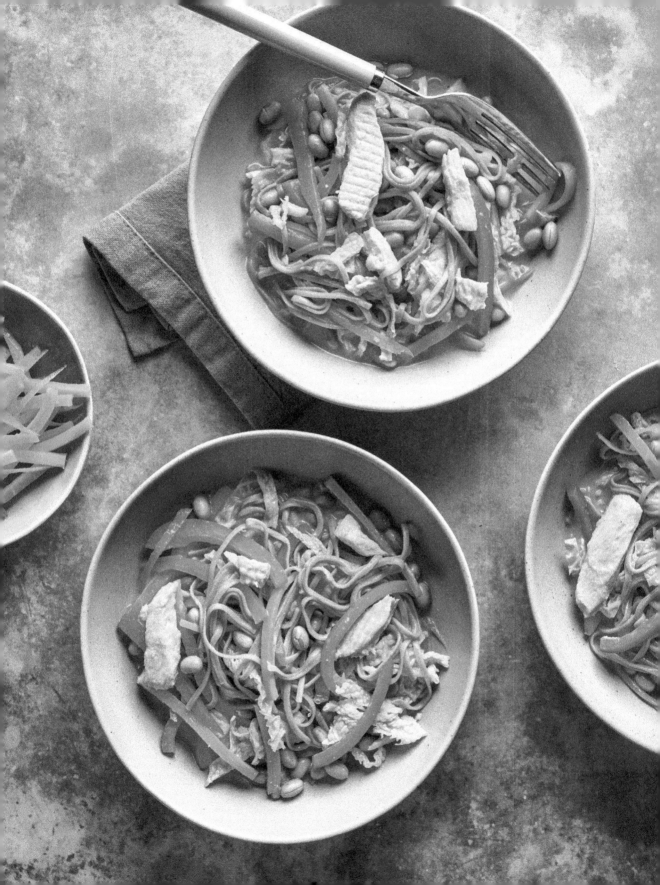

6

Poultry and Meat Entrees

While animal proteins can be a part of a healthy diet, it is recommended to limit intake of these foods. Many of these recipes can be made with plant proteins such as beans or tofu.

‹ Chicken and Veggie Soba Noodles, page 97

Rotisserie Chicken Noodle Soup

DIABETES-FRIENDLY • MEDIUM-PROTEIN • ONE POT

SERVES 6 • **PREP TIME:** 10 minutes • **COOK TIME:** 30 minutes

Chicken noodle soup is definitely one of my favorite comfort foods. This recipe uses a premade rotisserie chicken for easy cooking. You can also make your own chicken at home, which will definitely lower the sodium content of the recipe. You can have this as a meal as is or decrease the portion size to 6 to 8 ounces to have it as an appetizer with another meal.

8 cups no-salt-added or low-sodium chicken broth

1 cup chopped white onion

9 ounces rotisserie chicken, deboned and shredded

8 ounces elbow macaroni

1 cup chopped celery

1 cup chopped carrots

¼ teaspoon freshly ground black pepper

1. In a large soup pot, bring the chicken broth and onion to a boil over high heat.

2. Add the chicken, macaroni, celery, carrots, and pepper to the pot and bring back to a boil. Cook until the noodles are done, about 15 minutes.

3. Serve immediately.

4. Store leftovers in an airtight container in the refrigerator for up to 5 days. If you want to freeze, I recommend portioning out in individual servings or placing in a large resealable bag and laying flat in freezer to save space. Freeze for up to 3 months.

MAKE IT HEART-HEALTHY: Some rotisserie chicken may have high sodium content; rinse the meat under running water before placing it in the broth.

MAKE IT LOWER IN PROTEIN: Use less chicken in the broth or swap out the noodles for a lower-protein one, such as those from Flavis (see Resources page 148).

PER SERVING (2 CUPS): Calories: 281; Protein: 19.6g; Carbohydrates: 35g; Fiber: 3g; Total Fat: 7g; Saturated Fat: 2g; Sodium: 209mg; Cholesterol: 44mg; Potassium: 227mg; Phosphorus: 19mg

Chicken and Veggie Soba Noodles

DIABETES-FRIENDLY • HEART-HEALTHY • HIGH-PROTEIN

SERVES 4 • PREP TIME: 10 minutes • **COOK TIME:** 10 minutes

Soba noodles are made from buckwheat flour, which is very nutritious. These noodles are high in soluble fiber, which is good for your digestive and cardiovascular health, and it can also help with blood sugar management. These noodles are extremely versatile and can be eaten cold or hot! (Make sure to purchase noodles that are lower in sodium.)

6 ounces uncooked soba noodles

2 cups no-salt-added or low-sodium chicken broth

2 cups chopped green cabbage

1 medium red bell pepper, julienned

1 cup julienned carrots

1 cup frozen shelled edamame, thawed

1 (5-ounce) can Wild Planet no-salt-added chicken, drained and rinsed

½ cup Peanut Apple Sauce (page 141)

1 to 2 tablespoons water (optional)

1. In a large pot, heat the soba noodles and broth over high heat. Add the cabbage, bell pepper, and carrots.

2. Bring to a boil and cover the pot. Reduce the heat to low and simmer, stirring occasionally, for 5 to 7 minutes, until the noodles are cooked through and the vegetables are soft.

3. Remove from the heat. Add the edamame, chicken, and peanut apple sauce and toss together until mixed and evenly coated. You may want to add water if the mixture is too thick.

4. Store in an airtight container in the refrigerator for up to 5 days or in the freezer for up to 3 months.

MAKE IT LOWER IN PROTEIN: Leave out or cut the portion of chicken or edamame to reduce the protein content in the recipe and add more veggies instead.

PER SERVING (1½ CUPS): Calories: 369; Protein: 25.6g; Carbohydrates: 44g; Fiber: 7g; Total Fat: 12g; Saturated Fat: 2g; Sodium: 233mg; Cholesterol: 6mg; Potassium: 295mg; Phosphorus: 33mg

Jerk Chicken with Rice and Vegetables

DIABETES-FRIENDLY • MEDIUM-PROTEIN

SERVES 6 • **PREP TIME:** 15 minutes, plus 3 hours to chill • **COOK TIME:** 25 minutes

Jerk chicken is a popular dish from Jamaica. This recipe is the perfect example to show how spices and seasonings can give so much flavor. This dish is fragrant with smoky and spicy flavors and packs so much punch that you don't need to season the rice or vegetables.

1 small red onion, chopped

6 scallions, both white and green parts, chopped

2 habanero chile peppers, seeded and chopped

2 tablespoons white vinegar or lemon juice

2 tablespoons brown sugar or honey

1 tablespoon coconut aminos

1 tablespoon avocado oil

1 tablespoon minced fresh ginger

2 garlic cloves, minced

2 teaspoons chopped fresh thyme

1 teaspoon ground allspice

½ teaspoon salt

1. In a food processor, combine the onion, scallions, habanero, vinegar, brown sugar, coconut aminos, oil, ginger, garlic, thyme, allspice, salt, black pepper, nutmeg, and cinnamon. Puree until smooth.

2. Put the chicken in a large resealable bag and cover with the pureed sauce mixture.

3. Seal the bag and refrigerate for at least 3 hours or overnight.

4. Heat a grill to medium-high heat, spray with cooking spray, and add the marinated chicken thighs. Grill until the chicken is cooked through and reaches an internal temperature of 165°F.

5. Meanwhile, prepare the brown rice and steam the frozen vegetables according to the package instructions.

6. Remove from the grill and serve each thigh with ½ cup of brown rice and ½ cup of steamed vegetables.

½ teaspoon freshly
ground black pepper

¼ teaspoon
ground nutmeg

⅛ teaspoon ground
cinnamon

Avocado or olive oil
cooking spray

12 ounces boneless,
skinless chicken thighs

3 cups cooked
brown rice

3 cups frozen mixed
vegetables

7. Store leftovers in an airtight container in the refrigerator for up to 3 days and in the freezer for up to 3 months.

MAKE IT HEART-HEALTHY: Leave out the salt to lower the sodium content in this recipe. The nutrition content may vary depending on how much sauce you consume.

PER SERVING (2 OUNCES CHICKEN THIGH + ½ CUP BROWN RICE + ½ CUP STEAMED VEGETABLES): Calories: 301; Protein: 15.1g; Carbohydrates: 45g; Fiber: 7g; Total Fat: 7g; Saturated Fat: 1g; Sodium: 260mg; Cholesterol: 46mg; Potassium: 337mg; Phosphorus: 163mg

Sweet Soy Chicken Stir-Fry

DIABETES-FRIENDLY • HEART-HEALTHY • MEDIUM-PROTEIN

SERVES 2 • PREP TIME: 10 minutes • **COOK TIME:** 20 minutes

This quick stir-fry recipe is easy to make ahead and stores well. You can double the recipe to save more for later or to have as a healthy freezer meal ready for you on days you don't want to cook. You can adjust the brown rice portion depending on your carbohydrate needs, and be sure to purchase coconut aminos with no added sodium.

⅓ cup brown rice or 1 cup cooked brown rice

1 tablespoon coconut aminos

1 tablespoon red pepper flakes

2 teaspoons honey

2 teaspoons rice wine vinegar

1 teaspoon cornstarch, dissolved in 2 teaspoons water

2 garlic cloves, minced

4 ounces boneless, skinless chicken breast, cut into ½-inch cubes

1 tablespoon sesame oil, divided

6 cups frozen stir-fry vegetable mix

1. Cook the brown rice according to the package instructions and set aside.

2. In a medium bowl, whisk the coconut aminos, red pepper flakes, honey, vinegar, cornstarch mixture, and garlic. Add the chicken and mix together until well coated.

3. In a large wok or pan, heat ½ tablespoon of sesame oil over medium-high heat. Add the chicken and cook for 5 to 7 minutes, until browned and heated through.

4. Add the remaining ½ tablespoon of sesame oil and the vegetable mix. Cook for 5 to 7 minutes, until warmed through but still firm. You can cook the vegetables for longer if you prefer them softer.

5. Portion out ½ cup of brown rice and ½ of the chicken and veggie mixture. Serve immediately.

6. Store leftovers in an airtight container in the refrigerator for up to 3 days or in the freezer for up to 3 months.

PER SERVING (½ CUP BROWN RICE + ½ OF VEGGIE AND CHICKEN MIX): Calories: 362; Protein: 18.8g; Carbohydrates: 54g; Fiber: 8g; Total Fat: 9g; Saturated Fat: 2g; Sodium: 267mg; Cholesterol: 44mg; Potassium: 291mg; Phosphorus: 217mg

Turkey Flatbread Pizza

DIABETES-FRIENDLY • HEART-HEALTHY • MEDIUM-PROTEIN

SERVES 1 • PREP TIME: 5 minutes • **COOK TIME:** 15 minutes

Lavash is a thin flatbread that has Middle Eastern roots. It is a delicious option in place of breads and other higher-sodium grain products. You can use it for sandwich wraps, pizza crusts, and quesadillas. I enjoy using Atoria's Family Bakery lavash flatbread because they use simple ingredients and keep well in the refrigerator or freezer.

1 package Atoria's Family Bakery lavash flatbread

1 tablespoon no-salt-added tomato paste

1 teaspoon Italian Seasoning Blend (page 136)

1 ounce no-salt-added or low-sodium sliced turkey

1 large mushroom, thinly sliced

1 small zucchini, thinly sliced

1 mini red bell pepper, thinly sliced

½ cup chopped fresh baby kale

2 tablespoons grated low-sodium mozzarella cheese

1. Preheat the oven to 350°F.

2. Put the flatbread on a baking sheet or pizza pan. Spread with the tomato paste and sprinkle the Italian seasoning on top.

3. Add the turkey, mushroom, zucchini, bell pepper, and kale. Top with the cheese and bake for about 15 minutes, until the cheese is melted and the veggies are softened and warm.

4. Store leftovers in an airtight container in the refrigerator for up to 5 days.

MAKE IT SIMPLER: If you are unable to find Atoria's lavash flatbread in stores, you can check out their website and order it online. Alternatively, you can browse your local grocery store to find another flatbread, but be sure to compare food labels to make sure you find a product that fits your nutrition needs.

PER SERVING (1 PIZZA): Calories: 239; Protein: 19.4g; Carbohydrates: 31g; Fiber: 7g; Total Fat: 4g; Saturated Fat: 2g; Sodium: 189mg; Cholesterol: 29mg; Potassium: 579mg; Phosphorus: 141mg

Spicy Turkey Burgers

DIABETES-FRIENDLY • HIGH-PROTEIN

SERVES 5 • **PREP TIME:** 10 minutes • **COOK TIME:** 30 minutes

Turkey burgers are a great alternative to the typical beef burgers. They are lower in fat and just as delicious. This recipe is a bit on the spicy side, but you could use some basil or thyme instead of the red pepper flakes.

Avocado or olive oil cooking spray

12 ounces lean ground turkey

1 cup shredded zucchini

1 cup minced yellow onion

¼ cup panko bread crumbs

1 large egg

1 jalapeño pepper, seeded and minced

1 teaspoon red pepper flakes

½ teaspoon freshly ground black pepper

½ teaspoon garlic powder

2 medium poblano peppers, seeded and halved lengthwise

5 teaspoons Low-Sodium Dijon Mustard (page 139) or store-bought (optional)

5 whole-wheat hamburger buns

5 romaine lettuce leaves

1. Preheat the oven to 400°F. Line a baking sheet with foil and spray lightly with cooking spray.

2. In a large mixing bowl, combine the turkey, zucchini, onion, bread crumbs, egg, jalapeño, red pepper flakes, black pepper, and garlic powder. Mix until well combined.

3. Divide the meat mixture into 4 equal parts and form into 4 burger patties. Put the patties and poblano peppers on the prepared baking sheet. Bake for 20 to 25 minutes, until the patties are no longer pink and are cooked through to an internal temperature of 165°F.

4. Spread 1 teaspoon of mustard (if using) onto the bottom bun. Add 1 leaf of romaine, the turkey patty, and ½ a poblano pepper before placing the top bun. Serve immediately.

5. Store leftover patties in an airtight container in the refrigerator for up to 5 days. Store between parchment paper in an airtight container in the freezer for up to 3 months.

MAKE IT HEART-HEALTHY: Buy extra-lean (99 percent) ground turkey to lower the saturated fat content of this recipe. If you do use extra lean, add ½ tablespoon of olive oil to the recipe.

PER SERVING (1 BURGER): Calories: 279; Protein: 24g; Carbohydrates: 23g; Fiber: 2g; Total Fat: 10g; Saturated Fat: 3g; Sodium: 222mg; Cholesterol: 108mg; Potassium: 500mg; Phosphorus: 249mg

Turkey Nuggets with Roasted Vegetables

DIABETES-FRIENDLY • HEART-HEALTHY • MEDIUM-PROTEIN

SERVES 2 • **PREP TIME:** 10 minutes • **COOK TIME:** 25 minutes

These nuggets are made with lean turkey breast and are a great alternative to store-bought or restaurant nuggets. Swap up the flavors by trying different types of spices and seasoning.

1 small zucchini, cut into long strips

1 medium carrot, cut into long strips

1 small leek, cut into long strips

1 medium red bell pepper, cut into long strips

½ small eggplant, cut into long strips

1 small bunch broccolini

8 asparagus spears, trimmed

Avocado or olive oil cooking spray

¼ cup whole-grain panko bread crumbs

1 teaspoon Italian Seasoning Blend (page 136)

1 tablespoon olive or avocado oil, divided

5 ounces boneless, skinless turkey breast, diced

½ cup cooked brown lentils (if using canned lentils be sure to rinse and drain before using)

1. Preheat the oven to 400°F. Line a baking sheet with parchment paper.

2. Spread out the zucchini, carrots, leek, bell pepper, eggplant, broccolini, and asparagus on the baking sheet and lightly spray with cooking spray. Bake for about 25 minutes, until the vegetables are tender and lightly browned.

3. Meanwhile, in a medium bowl, mix together the bread crumbs, Italian seasoning, and ½ tablespoon of oil. Coat the turkey with the breadcrumb mixture and set aside.

4. In a medium pan, heat the remaining ½ tablespoon of oil over medium-high heat. Add the turkey nuggets and lightly fry for 5 to 8 minutes on each side, until golden brown and cooked through to an internal temperature of 165°F.

5. In a large bowl, add ¼ cup of lentils, half of the roasted vegetables, and half of the turkey nuggets. Serve immediately and enjoy!

6. Store leftovers in an airtight container in the refrigerator for up to 5 days and in the freezer for up to 3 months.

MAKE IT SIMPLER: Use a mandoline or food processor with a slicing attachment to evenly and quickly cut all the vegetables. Also, you can find precooked lentils and microwavable rice packets at most grocery stores.

PER SERVING (¼ CUP LENTILS + HALF THE VEGETABLES AND TURKEY NUGGETS): Calories: 287; Protein: 18.7g; Carbohydrates: 38g; Fiber: 8g; Total Fat: 8g; Saturated Fat: 1g; Sodium: 124mg; Cholesterol: 26mg; Potassium: 747mg; Phosphorus: 138mg

Turkey-Stuffed Bell Peppers

DIABETES-FRIENDLY • HEART-HEALTHY • HIGH-PROTEIN

SERVES 4 • **PREP TIME:** 5 minutes • **COOK TIME:** 40 minutes

Bell peppers are a delicious fruit that can be used as a vessel for many different recipes. They are nutritious and low in calories. Bell peppers come in a range of colors—red, yellow, orange, and green, with red being the most sweet and green a bit more bitter. These fruits are packed with vitamin C and antioxidants. Use a ground turkey that is at least 95 percent lean for this recipe.

1 tablespoon avocado oil

8 ounces lean ground turkey

½ cup finely chopped yellow onion

1 cup grated carrots

½ teaspoon garlic powder

½ teaspoon Italian Seasoning Blend (page 136)

¼ teaspoon paprika

2 cups cooked white rice

2 medium bell peppers, any color, halved lengthwise

2 tablespoons grated Parmesan cheese

1. Preheat the oven to 400°F.

2. In a medium pan or skillet, heat the oil over medium heat. Add the turkey, onion, carrots, garlic powder, Italian seasoning, and paprika. Sauté for 4 to 5 minutes, until the meat is cooked through.

3. Add the cooked rice and cook for another 2 minutes.

4. Put the sliced bell pepper halves into a baking dish. Scoop one-quarter of the meat mixture (about ¾ cup) into each pepper half and top each with ½ tablespoon of Parmesan cheese.

5. Bake for 25 to 30 minutes until the peppers have softened. Serve immediately and enjoy!

6. Store cooled leftovers in an airtight container in the refrigerator for up to 4 days.

PER SERVING (½ BELL PEPPER): Calories: 307; Protein: 19.6g; Carbohydrates: 32g; Fiber: 2g; Total Fat: 11g; Saturated Fat: 3g; Sodium: 129mg; Cholesterol: 62mg; Potassium: 440mg; Phosphorus: 232mg

Lemon-Rosemary Pork with Cauliflower Mash

DIABETES-FRIENDLY • HEART-HEALTHY • HIGH-PROTEIN

SERVES 4 • **PREP TIME:** 5 minutes • **COOK TIME:** 10 minutes

This is a quick and easy meal that you can whip up during your busy week. Make your cauliflower mash ahead of time and have it ready to pair with this meal for an even faster meal prep. Increase or decrease the amount of pork depending on each family member's needs.

2 tablespoons all-purpose flour

1 teaspoon freshly ground black pepper

12 ounces pork cutlets, fat trimmed

2 teaspoons avocado oil

1 cup freshly squeezed lemon juice

¼ cup no-salt-added or low-sodium chicken broth

1 tablespoon coarsely chopped fresh rosemary

2 cups Cauliflower Mash (page 63)

2 cups carrot sticks, raw or steamed

Rosemary sprigs, for garnish (optional)

1. In a shallow dish, combine the flour and pepper. Lightly coat the pork in the mixture.

2. In a large skillet or pan, heat the oil over medium-high heat. Add the pork and cook for 2 to 3 minutes per side, or until golden brown on each side and no longer pink in the middle.

3. Remove from the pan and cover with foil. Set aside. In the same pan, increase the heat to high and combine the lemon juice, broth, and rosemary. Stir occasionally and bring to a boil for about 3 to 4 minutes. The sauce should be slightly thickened.

4. Arrange 2 to 3 ounces of pork on a plate and serve with ½ cup of cauliflower mash and ½ cup of carrot sticks. Pour the lemon sauce over the pork, garnish with rosemary (if using), and serve immediately.

5. Store leftovers in an airtight container in the refrigerator for up to 5 days and in the freezer for up to 3 months.

PER SERVING (2 OUNCES PORK + ½ CUP CAULIFLOWER MASHED "POTATOES" + ½ CUP CARROT STICKS): Calories: 286; Protein: 21.9g; Carbohydrates: 20g; Fiber: 6g; Total Fat: 14g; Saturated Fat: 5g; Sodium: 198mg; Cholesterol: 61mg; Potassium: 657mg; Phosphorus: 236mg

Baked Apple Pork Chops with Wild Rice and Green Beans

DIABETES-FRIENDLY • HEART-HEALTHY • HIGH-PROTEIN

SERVES 4 • PREP TIME: 10 minutes • **COOK TIME:** 1 hour

This dish may have a longer cooking time, but most of that is spent with it in the oven. The pork chops in this recipe are juicy, tender, and sweet. Trim the fat from the pork chops to avoid any unnecessary unhealthy saturated fats. You can easily adapt this recipe with different types of proteins and swap out the veggies for whatever is your favorite.

Avocado or olive oil cooking spray

2 tablespoons avocado or olive oil

9 ounces center loin pork chops

2 medium apples, cored and sliced

1 pound green beans, trimmed

½ cup water

2 tablespoons brown sugar or honey

2 tablespoons apple cider vinegar

½ teaspoon salt

½ teaspoon freshly ground black pepper

1 cup cooked wild rice

1. Preheat the oven to 325°F. Line an oven-safe pan with foil and spray with cooking spray.

2. In a medium skillet or pan, heat the oil over medium-high heat. Add the pork chops and brown on each side for 2 to 3 minutes. Remove from the pan and place in the prepared oven pan and top with the sliced apples. Add the green beans to the pan in a single layer and lightly spray with cooking spray.

3. Deglaze the skillet with the water, stirring to scrape up the browned bits from the bottom. Pour the mixture over the pork chops and green beans.

4. Sprinkle the brown sugar, vinegar, salt, and pepper over the pork chops. Cover the pan with foil and bake for about 30 minutes. Uncover and cook for an additional 15 to 20 minutes. Meanwhile, heat the wild rice in the microwave until hot.

5. Serve the pork with the apples, green beans, and a side of rice.

6. Store leftovers in an airtight container in the refrigerator for up to 5 days and in the freezer for up to 3 months.

MAKE IT LOWER IN PROTEIN: Reduce the portion of your pork depending on your protein needs and instead increase the amount of green beans or wild rice to add more substance to your meal.

PER SERVING (¼ CUP WILD RICE + ½ CUP GREEN BEANS + 2 OUNCES PORK): Calories: 305; Protein: 20.1g; Carbohydrates: 35g; Fiber: 7g; Total Fat: 11g; Saturated Fat: 2g; Sodium: 338mg; Cholesterol: 43mg; Potassium: 562mg; Phosphorus: 244mg

Spiced Lamb Meatballs with Roasted Vegetables

DIABETES-FRIENDLY • HIGH-PROTEIN

SERVES 5 • **PREP TIME:** 10 minutes • **COOK TIME:** 40 minutes

This is another recipe that looks quite complicated but is very simple and easy to make. The majority of ingredients consist of spices that make this dish tasty and fragrant without any added salt. This dish freezes well and can easily be made ahead of time.

FOR THE VEGETABLES

1 medium head cauliflower, cut into florets

2 cups carrots, cut into medallions

2 tablespoons avocado or olive oil

1 teaspoon ground cumin

½ teaspoon ground cinnamon

½ teaspoon paprika

¼ teaspoon freshly ground black pepper

1¼ cups frozen corn

FOR THE MEATBALLS

1 pound ground lamb

¼ cup whole-wheat bread crumbs

1 large egg, lightly beaten

1 teaspoon garlic powder or 1 garlic clove, minced

TO MAKE THE VEGETABLES

1. Preheat the oven to 400°F.

2. Line a baking pan with parchment paper and spread out the cauliflower and carrots in a single layer. Drizzle with oil and sprinkle with cumin, cinnamon, paprika, and black pepper and toss to coat. Roast for 20 to 25 minutes until lightly browned.

TO MAKE THE MEATBALLS

3. Meanwhile, in a large mixing bowl, combine the lamb, bread crumbs, egg, garlic powder, coriander, cumin, paprika, cinnamon, black pepper, and cayenne (if using) and mix until combined. Do not overwork the meat or it will be tough. Roll into 1-inch balls.

4. Once the vegetables have cooked for 20 to 25 minutes, flip them over and add the meatballs to the pan. Nestle the meatballs between the vegetables and put the pan back in the oven. Bake for 15 minutes until cooked through.

½ teaspoon ground coriander

½ teaspoon ground cumin

½ teaspoon paprika

½ teaspoon ground cinnamon

½ teaspoon freshly ground black pepper

½ teaspoon ground cayenne pepper (optional)

FOR THE MINT TAHINI SAUCE

¼ cup tahini

3 to 4 tablespoons warm water

2 tablespoons finely chopped fresh mint or 1 tablespoon dried mint

Freshly squeezed lemon juice

TO MAKE THE MINT TAHINI SAUCE

5. Meanwhile, in a small bowl, combine the tahini, water, mint, and lemon juice to taste.

6. Heat up the corn according to the package instructions, then toss with the vegetable and meatball mixture.

7. When the food is done cooking, divide into 4 equal portions and drizzle the sauce on top.

8. Store leftovers in an airtight container in the refrigerator for up to 5 days and in the freezer for up to 3 months. The sauce can be stored in the refrigerator, but I don't recommend freezing. When ready to reheat frozen food, make the sauce.

MAKE IT HEART-HEALTHY: Use lean lamb meat or substitute it with your favorite lean poultry, such as chicken or turkey.

PER SERVING (3 MEATBALLS + ½ CUP VEGETABLES + ¼ CUP CORN): Calories: 436; Protein: 24.7g; Carbohydrates: 26g; Fiber: 8g; Total Fat: 28g; Saturated Fat: 8g; Sodium: 150mg; Cholesterol: 103mg; Potassium: 747mg; Phosphorus: 341mg

Sweet and Sour Beef Meatballs

DIABETES-FRIENDLY • HEART-HEALTHY • MEDIUM-PROTEIN

SERVES 10 • PREP TIME: 10 minutes **• COOK TIME:** 20 minutes

I love all things that are sweet and sour, and this recipe is a fun twist on a popular dish. These meatballs are sure to be a hit with everyone of all ages and they are a great way to sneak in some vegetables for those who aren't so keen on them. Try this easy recipe with any of your favorite meat or protein.

FOR THE MEATBALLS

2 pounds extra-lean ground beef

½ cup diced zucchini

½ cup diced carrots

½ cup diced orange bell pepper

½ cup diced yellow onion

¼ cup plain Unsweetened Almond Milk (page 143), or store-bought

1 tablespoon low-sodium soy sauce

1 tablespoon low-sodium Worcestershire sauce

1 garlic clove, minced

¼ teaspoon ground cinnamon

FOR THE SAUCE

1 cup water

⅓ cup apple cider vinegar

¼ cup packed brown sugar

TO MAKE THE MEATBALLS

1. Preheat the oven to 375°F and line a baking sheet with parchment paper. Set aside.

2. In a large bowl, combine the beef, zucchini, carrots, bell pepper, onion, almond milk, soy sauce, Worcestershire sauce, garlic, and cinnamon and mix until combined. Do not overwork the meat or it will be tough.

3. Roll into 1-inch balls and put on the prepared baking sheet. Bake until the meatballs are cooked through, about 15 minutes.

TO MAKE THE SAUCE

4. Meanwhile, in a large stockpot, combine the water, vinegar, brown sugar, cornstarch, soy sauce, and sesame oil and mix until well combined. Turn the heat to medium-low and bring the mixture to a simmer, stirring occasionally, for about 5 minutes, until the sauce thickens. Add the pineapple chunks and toss to coat. When the meatballs are done cooking, add them to the sauce and mix to coat.

5. To serve, plate ½ cup of rice and 5 meatballs.

6 tablespoons cornstarch

2 tablespoons low-sodium soy sauce

½ teaspoon sesame oil

1 (40-ounce) can pineapple chunks in 100 percent juice, (reserve 1½ cups pineapple juice)

2 cups cooked white or brown rice, for serving

6. Store leftovers in an airtight container in the refrigerator for up to 5 days and in the freezer for up to 3 months.

MAKE IT SIMPLER: Use a food processor to chop the vegetables to cut down on prep time and manual labor.

PER SERVING (5 MEATBALLS + ½ CUP RICE):
Calories: 294; Protein: 20.1g; Carbohydrates: 46g; Fiber: 2g; Total Fat: 4g; Saturated Fat: 2g; Sodium: 202mg; Cholesterol: 60mg; Potassium: 544mg; Phosphorus: 184mg

Taco-Seasoned Roast Beef Wraps

DIABETES-FRIENDLY • MEDIUM-PROTEIN

SERVES 2 • PREP TIME: 10 minutes

This meal can be whipped up quickly for those busy days. It is convenient to eat and can be taken to go! These wraps can also be made with other types of protein such as chicken, turkey, or tofu.

2 tablespoons low-fat cream cheese

2 (10-inch) flour tortillas

1 teaspoon Taco Seasoning (page 134)

4 ounces low-sodium roast beef

½ cup fresh spinach

2 tablespoons diced red onion

2 tablespoons pimento or cherry pepper, halved lengthwise

1. Spread 1 tablespoon of cream cheese on 1 tortilla and sprinkle the taco seasoning on top.

2. Add 2 ounces of roast beef and top with ¼ cup of spinach, 1 tablespoon of red onion, and 1 tablespoon of pimento pepper.

3. Roll up and enjoy!

MAKE IT HEART-HEALTHY: Instead of using processed deli meat, make your own roast beef without salt at home and slice it. This will lower the sodium content significantly. You can also try checking your local deli to see whether they have a low-sodium or no-salt-added roast beef.

PER SERVING (1 WRAP): Calories: 289; Protein: 19.6g; Carbohydrates: 27g; Fiber: 1g; Total Fat: 11g; Saturated Fat: 4g; Sodium: 432mg; Cholesterol: 49mg; Potassium: 256mg; Phosphorus: 21mg

Chili with Flatbread Crackers

DIABETES-FRIENDLY • HIGH-PROTEIN

SERVES 4 • **PREP TIME:** 5 minutes • **COOK TIME:** 1 hour 10 minutes

Cut the cooking time by using a pressure cooker to make this chili; simply select the sauté function to cook the beef and onion, add the remaining ingredients, mix together, and secure the lid. Pressure cook on high pressure for 10 minutes and let it release naturally for 15 minutes. Use Wasa multigrain crispbread or Milton's crackers.

1 tablespoon avocado or olive oil

8 ounces extra-lean ground beef

1 large onion, diced

2 cups no-salt-added or low-sodium beef broth

2 cups no-salt-added canned tomato sauce

1 medium red bell pepper, diced

1 (4-ounce) can green chili peppers, drained, rinsed, and diced

2 tablespoons chili powder

1 tablespoon garlic powder

1 teaspoon dried basil

½ teaspoon dried oregano

½ teaspoon dried thyme

¼ teaspoon ground cumin

16 Garlic and Herb Flatbread Crackers (page 128) or store-bought

1. In a large stockpot, cook the ground beef over medium heat for about 5 minutes until browned.

2. Add the onion and cook for about 3 minutes until soft.

3. Add the broth, tomato sauce, bell pepper, chili peppers, chili powder, garlic powder, basil, oregano, thyme, and cumin and stir until well combined. Bring the pot to a boil and reduce the heat to medium-low. Simmer for an hour.

4. Serve 1 cup of chili with 4 flatbread crackers.

5. Store leftovers in an airtight container in the refrigerator for up to 5 days and in the freezer for up to 3 months.

MAKE IT LOWER IN PROTEIN: If your protein needs are lower, decrease the amount of beef you use in the recipe or try swapping out the beef for kidney beans and use a low-sodium vegetable broth.

PER SERVING (1 CUP CHILI + 4 CRACKERS): Calories: 303; Protein: 20.6g; Carbohydrates: 27g; Fiber: 3g; Total Fat: 13g; Saturated Fat: 3g; Sodium: 343mg; Cholesterol: 50mg; Potassium: 685mg; Phosphorus: 181mg

Beef Shish Kebabs with Grilled Corn

DIABETES-FRIENDLY • HEART-HEALTHY • HIGH-PROTEIN

SERVES 6 • PREP TIME: 10 minutes, plus 1 hour
to marinate • **COOK TIME:** 10 minutes

This recipe is another quick and easy meal that is packed with flavors and customizable to your specific tastes. Try it with some of the seasoning blends from chapter 8 (page 133).

½ cup apple
cider vinegar

½ cup olive or
avocado oil

½ teaspoon freshly
ground black pepper

½ teaspoon
dried oregano

¼ teaspoon
garlic powder

1 pound beef sirloin, cut
into 1½-inch cubes

2 medium white onions,
quartered

2 medium green bell
peppers, cut into
1½-inch squares

1 medium red bell
pepper, cut into
1½-inch squares

6 medium corn cobs,
husks and silks removed

1. In a large bowl, combine the vinegar, olive oil, black pepper, oregano, and garlic powder.

2. Add the sirloin, onions, and bell peppers to the bowl and mix to evenly coat. Cover the bowl with plastic wrap, put in the refrigerator, and let marinate for 1 hour. If using wooden skewers, soak them in water for 30 minutes.

3. Load the skewers with the meat and chopped vegetables, alternating pieces of the sirloin, bell peppers, and corn. Grill the kebabs and corn over medium heat. Cook the kebabs for 4 to 5 minutes on each side. Cooking times can be adjusted based on how well you like the meat cooked. Cook the corn for about 10 minutes, turning often. Serve immediately.

4. Leftovers can be stored in the refrigerator in airtight containers for up to 5 days.

MAKE IT SIMPLER: You can also bake these kebabs in the oven. Preheat the oven to 350°F. You will cook the kebabs for about 30 minutes and turn them every 10 minutes. Wrap the corn in foil and bake for 20 to 25 minutes, turning once halfway through.

PER SERVING (1 KEBAB + 1 CORN COB): Calories: 381; Protein: 21.3g; Carbohydrates: 28g; Fiber: 4g; Total Fat: 22g; Saturated Fat: 3g; Sodium: 42mg; Cholesterol: 44mg; Potassium: 586mg; Phosphorus: 253mg

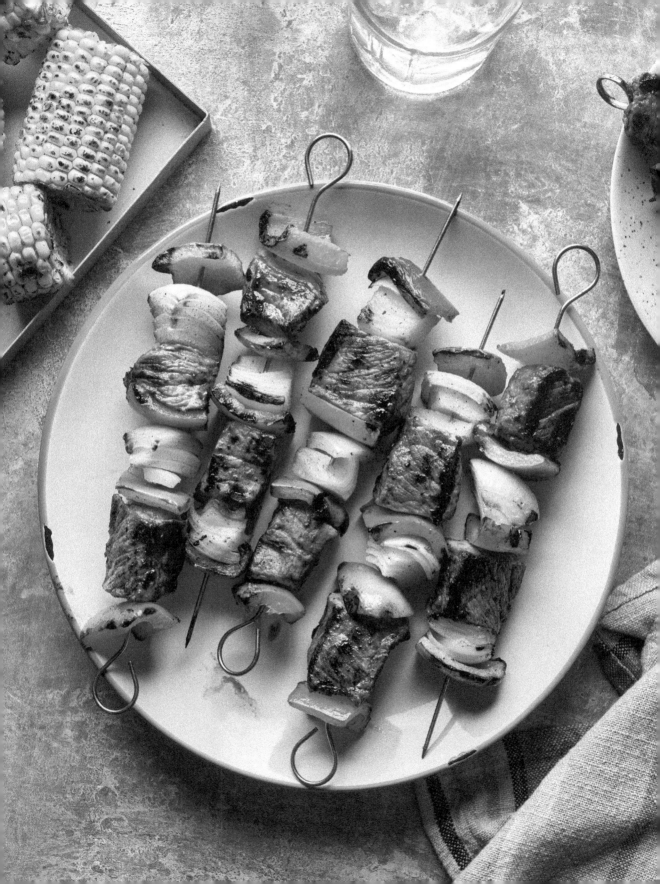

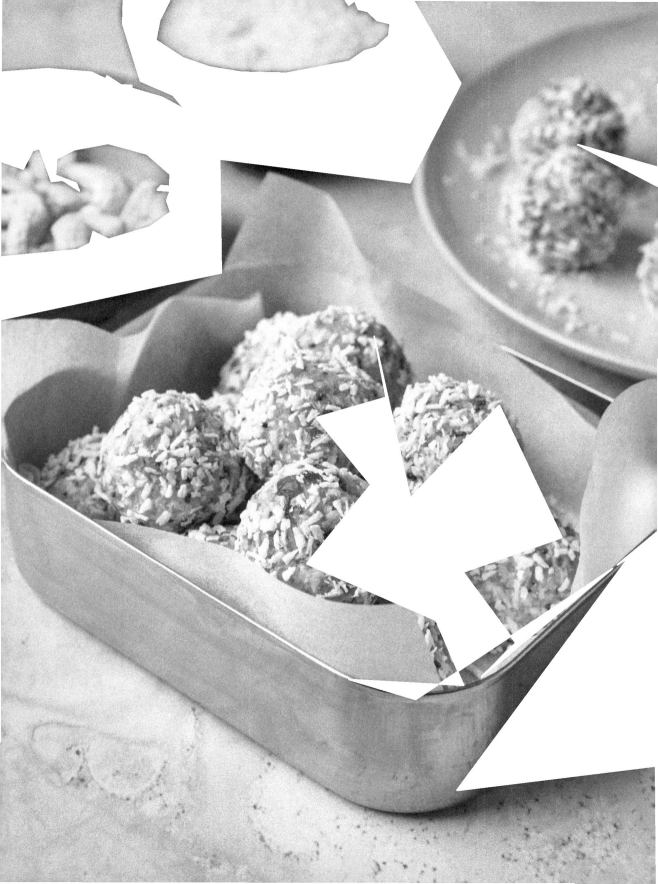

7

Sweets and Snacks

◁ Tangy Lemon Energy Bites, page 123

Cucumber Pineapple Cooler

DIABETES-FRIENDLY • HEART-HEALTHY • LOW-PROTEIN
ONE POT • 5 INGREDIENTS OR FEWER

SERVES 2 • PREP TIME: 5 minutes

A refreshing drink that's low in calories, protein, and fat, this beverage is perfect for a warm summer day or an afternoon refresher. This is also a perfect way to flavor your water if you aren't a fan of plain.

2 medium cucumbers, peeled and sliced

2 cups water (regular or sparkling)

1 cup frozen pineapple chunks

1 cup ice

Mint leaves, for garnish

1. In a blender, combine the cucumbers, water, pineapple, and ice and blend until a slushy forms.

2. Divide between 2 glasses and garnish with mint leaves before serving.

MAKE IT SIMPLER: You can also create an infused water by putting all the ingredients into a pitcher and letting it sit for at least 15 minutes.

PER SERVING (1 CUP): Calories: 85; Protein: 2g; Carbohydrates: 19g; Fiber 3g; Total Fat: 0g; Saturated Fat: 0g; Sodium: 14mg; Cholesterol: 0mg; Potassium: 273mg; Phosphorus: 42mg

Raspberry Pear Sorbet

DIABETES-FRIENDLY • LOW-PROTEIN • 5 INGREDIENTS OR FEWER

SERVES 6 • **PREP TIME:** 5 minutes, plus 12 hours to freeze

This sorbet is a nice and refreshing treat that's perfect for hot summer days or as a treat after a meal. This version is a much better alternative with whole ingredients and fresh fruits. Add protein powder in step 2 to add a little bit more protein to balance out the meal. Alternatively, you can also omit the sugar to lower the carbohydrate content.

1 cup water

¼ cup granulated sugar

2 cups fresh or frozen raspberries

2 medium pears, peeled, cored, and sliced

⅓ cup freshly squeezed lime juice

1. In a small saucepan, combine the water and sugar and bring to a boil to dissolve the sugar. Reduce the heat and let simmer, uncovered, for 3 minutes to create a simple syrup. Remove from the heat and put in the refrigerator to cool.

2. In a food processor or blender, combine the raspberries, pears, and lime juice. Blend for 30 seconds to 1 minute, until the mixture is smooth. Add the cooled syrup and mix well.

3. Spread the mixture into a baking pan and cover with plastic wrap. Place in the freezer for 4 hours or until the mixture is solid. Using a fork, break the mixture into pieces and put it back in a food processor or blender and puree for 30 seconds. Transfer the mixture into a container, cover, and freeze again for 6 to 8 hours, or until solid. When ready to serve, let sit at room temperature for a few minutes before scooping.

4. Store leftovers in the freezer in a sealed container for up to 6 months.

PER SERVING (½ CUP): Calories: 97; Protein: 0.9g; Carbohydrates: 25g; Fiber: 5g; Total Fat: 0g; Saturated Fat: 0g; Sodium: 3mg; Cholesterol: 0mg; Potassium: 166mg; Phosphorus: 25mg

Dark Chocolate Chickpea Balls

DIABETES-FRIENDLY • HEART-HEALTHY • LOW-PROTEIN

SERVES 15 • **PREP TIME:** 5 minutes, plus 15 minutes to chill

I love chocolate and this recipe definitely hits the spot. These chickpea balls can be made ahead and stores well, so that you can always have a healthy fix for your chocolate craving. They're fun to make and can be enjoyed by the whole family.

1 (15-ounce) can no-salt-added chickpeas, drained, rinsed, and patted dry

⅓ cup oat flour

¼ cup creamy unsalted peanut butter

3 tablespoons maple syrup or honey

1 teaspoon vanilla extract

¼ teaspoon ground cinnamon

⅓ cup dark chocolate chips or cacao nibs

1. Line a baking sheet with parchment paper.

2. In a food processor, combine the chickpeas, oat flour, peanut butter, maple syrup, vanilla, and cinnamon. Process until a dough forms.

3. Scoop out the dough and knead in the chocolate chips until well incorporated. Roll into balls using a heaping tablespoon, about 1 inch in size, and put on the baking sheet. Leave in the refrigerator and let harden for at least 15 minutes.

4. Store leftovers in an airtight container in the refrigerator for up to 1 week or in the freezer for up to 6 months. If storing in the freezer, let defrost for 5 to 10 minutes before eating.

MAKE IT SIMPLER: Make your own oat flour by placing oats in a food processor or blender and blend until a fine flour consistency forms.

PER SERVING (1 BALL): Calories: 95; Protein: 2.8g; Carbohydrates: 11g; Fiber: 2g; Total Fat: 4g; Saturated Fat: 1g; Sodium: 5mg; Cholesterol: 0mg; Potassium: 38mg; Phosphorus: 13mg

Tangy Lemon Energy Bites

DIABETES-FRIENDLY • HEART-HEALTHY • LOW-PROTEIN

SERVES 18 • **PREP TIME:** 20 minutes

These no-bake energy bites are super easy to make and are full of healthy fats, tangy flavor, and are perfect as an afternoon pick-me-up snack. This recipe stores well and can be made ahead of time, so you always have a healthy snack on hand. Roll the finished bites in more shredded unsweetened coconut, if desired.

8 Medjool dates, pitted

1 cup raw unsalted cashews

1 cup unsweetened shredded coconut

2 tablespoons grated lemon zest

2 tablespoons freshly squeezed lemon juice

1 tablespoon chia seeds

½ teaspoon vanilla extract

1. Put the dates in a medium bowl and cover with hot water. Let soak for 15 minutes, then drain.

2. In a blender or food processor, pulse the cashews until finely chopped. Add the dates, coconut, lemon zest and juice, chia seeds, and vanilla and pulse until everything is well combined and a sticky dough forms.

3. Using a tablespoon, scoop out the dough and roll it into balls. If the dough doesn't form balls, add more lemon juice, 1 teaspoon at a time.

4. Store leftovers in the refrigerator for up to 1 week or in the freezer for up to 3 months. Let defrost for 5 to 10 minutes before eating if storing in the freezer.

PER SERVING (1 BITE): Calories: 102; Protein: 1.9g; Carbohydrates: 12g; Fiber: 2g; Total Fat: 6g; Saturated Fat: 3g; Sodium: 3mg; Cholesterol: 0mg; Potassium: 150mg; Phosphorus: 64mg

Carrot Cake Cookies

DIABETES-FRIENDLY • HEART-HEALTHY • LOW-PROTEIN

SERVES 15 • PREP TIME: 15 minutes • **COOK TIME:** 20 minutes

This recipe transforms the classic carrot cake into cookie form, which is great to help with portion control. It makes a ton of cookies and stores well in the freezer, so you can easily make this ahead of time and have it when you are craving a sweet treat.

1 cup all-purpose flour

1 cup rolled oats

2 teaspoons ground cinnamon

1 teaspoon ground ginger

1 teaspoon ground nutmeg

½ teaspoon baking powder

1 cup grated carrots

½ cup avocado or olive oil

¼ cup honey

1 large orange, zested

1. Preheat the oven to 350°F. Line a baking sheet with parchment paper and set aside.

2. In a large mixing bowl, combine the flour, oats, cinnamon, ginger, nutmeg, and baking powder.

3. Add the carrots, oil, and honey and mix until combined. Fold in the orange zest.

4. Scoop rounded teaspoons of batter onto the prepared baking sheet. Flatten the cookies to about ½-inch thick.

5. Bake for 15 to 20 minutes, until cooked through and the bottoms are lightly browned. Let sit for a couple minutes before transferring to a cooling rack. Serve warm or at room temperature.

6. Cookies can be stored in an airtight container in the refrigerator for up to 5 days or in the freezer for up to 6 months.

MAKE IT SIMPLER: You can purchase pre-grated carrots from your local supermarket to cut down on manual labor and prep time.

PER SERVING (2 COOKIES): Calories: 137; Protein: 1.7g; Carbohydrates: 16g; Fiber: 1g; Total Fat: 8g; Saturated Fat: 1g; Sodium: 22mg; Cholesterol: 0mg; Potassium: 59mg; Phosphorus: 38mg

Cinnamon Apple Chia Seed Pudding

HEART-HEALTHY • LOW-PROTEIN • ONE POT

SERVES 1 • PREP TIME: 5 minutes, plus 8 hours to set

This is a delicious sweet treat that you won't believe is healthy and packed with nutrients. Make it ahead of time for a grab-and-go snack. Add some peanut butter or protein powder to turn this into a meal. Customize this pudding with different fruits and toppings, like 1 tablespoon of chopped walnuts or sliced almonds—I also enjoy it with frozen strawberries and cacao nibs or bananas and peanut butter.

½ small unpeeled apple, chopped or grated

½ cup plain Unsweetened Almond Milk (page 143) or store-bought

2 tablespoons chia seeds

1 tablespoon maple syrup

¼ teaspoon vanilla extract

¼ teaspoon ground cinnamon

1. In a small bowl or 8-ounce mason jar, mix the apple, almond milk, chia seeds, maple syrup, vanilla, and cinnamon.

2. Cover and refrigerate overnight, or for at least 8 hours. When ready to enjoy, stir again.

3. Store in an airtight container in the refrigerator for up to 3 days.

MAKE IT DIABETES-FRIENDLY: Use ½ tablespoon of maple syrup to lower the carbohydrate content of this recipe.

PER SERVING (1 PUDDING CUP): Calories: 210; Protein: 4g; Carbohydrates: 34g; Fiber: 9g; Total Fat: 7g; Saturated Fat: 1g; Sodium: 93mg; Cholesterol: 0mg; Potassium: 288mg; Phosphorus: 192mg

PB Chocolate Fudge

DIABETES-FRIENDLY • HEART-HEALTHY • LOW-PROTEIN • ONE POT

MAKES 16 PIECES • **PREP TIME:** 5 minutes, plus 15 minutes to chill

This fudge is a delicious, ooey-gooey chocolatey treat. It's super easy to whip up and freezes well. This chocolate treat hits the spot when you are craving something decadent. Be sure to choose a nut butter and maple syrup that have minimal ingredients and no added salt or sugar.

¾ cup unsalted creamy peanut butter or nut butter of your choice

½ cup almond flour or oat flour

½ cup unsweetened cacao powder or cocoa powder

⅓ cup maple syrup

¼ cup dark chocolate chips

1 teaspoon vanilla extract

1 teaspoon ground cinnamon

1. Line an 8-by-8-inch baking pan with parchment paper.

2. In a large mixing bowl, combine the peanut butter, almond flour, cacao powder, maple syrup, chocolate chips, vanilla, and cinnamon and mix until well combined.

3. Pour the thick batter into the baking pan and put another sheet of parchment paper on top. Push down on the batter and spread evenly, until about ¼ to ½ inch in thickness.

4. Set in freezer for 15 minutes until hardened. Cut and serve.

5. Store leftovers in an airtight container in the freezer for up to 3 months. Let thaw slightly, 5 to 10 minutes, before eating.

PER SERVING (2-INCH SQUARE): Calories: 130; Protein: 3.8g; Carbohydrates: 10g; Fiber 2g; Total Fat: 9g; Saturated Fat: 2g; Sodium: 4mg; Cholesterol: 0mg; Potassium: 60mg; Phosphorus: 25mg

Open-Faced Turkey Crackers

DIABETES-FRIENDLY • HEART-HEALTHY • MEDIUM-PROTEIN • ONE POT

SERVES 2 • PREP TIME: 5 minutes

For this recipe, I enjoy using Wasa multigrain crispbread crackers, which are full of fiber and B vitamins, low in sodium, and have no added sugars. You can find these crackers at Walmart, Vons, and Sprouts. This recipe is also very customizable: Try it with chickpeas as your protein or layer with hummus. You can even make it a sweet snack by using plain unsweetened Greek yogurt and topping with some fresh fruit and a sprinkle of sliced almonds.

2 multigrain crispbread crackers

1 tablespoon Low-Sodium Dijon Mustard (page 139) or store-bought

2 ounces no-salt-added or low-sodium sliced turkey

½ small red bell pepper, thinly sliced

½ small cucumber, thinly sliced

½ cup fresh spinach

1. Lay a cracker on a plate. Spread ½ tablespoon of mustard on the cracker. Top with 1 ounce of turkey and half of the bell pepper, cucumber, and spinach.

2. Repeat for the second cracker. Enjoy!

PER SERVING (1 CRACKER): Calories: 152; Protein: 11.5g; Carbohydrates: 17g; Fiber: 4g; Total Fat 3g; Saturated Fat: 0g; Sodium: 123mg; Cholesterol: 20mg; Potassium: 315mg; Phosphorus: 77mg

Garlic and Herb Flatbread Crackers with Cilantro-Lime Yogurt Dip

DIABETES-FRIENDLY • HEART-HEALTHY • LOW-PROTEIN

SERVES 12 • **PREP TIME:** 10 minutes • **COOK TIME:** 20 minutes

Growing up, we always bought crackers and so I never knew how easy it is to make your own. These flatbread crackers are full of flavor and made without any preservatives or weird ingredients. I love that these can be customized by swapping out the seasonings! You can make this spicy by adding some red pepper flakes or sweet by using cinnamon and some sugar.

FOR THE CRACKERS

1¾ cups all-purpose flour, plus more for kneading

1½ tablespoons Mrs. Dash Garlic & Herb Seasoning Blend

2 teaspoons granulated sugar

½ cup water

⅓ cup olive oil

1 egg white or 2 tablespoons liquid egg whites

FOR THE CILANTRO-LIME YOGURT DIP

¾ cup plain nonfat Greek yogurt

2 tablespoons chopped fresh cilantro

1 tablespoon freshly squeezed lime juice

TO MAKE THE CRACKERS

1. Preheat the oven to 400°F. Line a baking sheet with parchment paper and set aside.

2. In a medium bowl, combine the flour, garlic and herb seasoning, and sugar and mix well.

3. Using a spoon, make a well in the dry ingredients and pour the water, oil, and egg white into the well. Mix together until the dough comes together. If the dough is too wet, add flour, 1 tablespoon at a time, until a drier dough forms.

4. Flour a flat work surface and knead the dough for 3 to 4 minutes. Divide the dough into four equal pieces and form each piece into a ball. Add more flour to the work surface and use a rolling pin dusted with flour to roll the dough ball very thin, about ⅛ inch.

5. Cut the dough into 12 squares or strips and evenly space on the prepared baking sheet. Use a fork to lightly pierce the dough.

6. Bake for 8 to 10 minutes, until the crackers are golden brown and crisp.

7. Repeat with each piece of dough, using a new sheet of parchment for each batch.

TO MAKE THE CILANTRO-LIME YOGURT DIP

8. Meanwhile, in a small bowl, mix the yogurt, cilantro, and lime juice until well combined. Serve 4 crackers with 1 tablespoon of dip.

9. Cooled crackers can be stored in an airtight container at room temperature for 3 days or in the refrigerator for up to 5 days. Store the dip in the refrigerator in an airtight container for up to 5 days.

PER SERVING (4 CRACKERS + 1 TABLESPOON DIP): Calories: 133; Protein: 3.8g; Carbohydrates: 15g; Fiber: 1g; Total Fat: 6g; Saturated Fat: 1g; Sodium: 11mg; Cholesterol: 1mg; Potassium: 53mg; Phosphorus: 41mg

Barbecue Roasted Chickpeas

DIABETES-FRIENDLY • LOW-PROTEIN • ONE POT • 5 INGREDIENTS OR FEWER

SERVES 6 • PREP TIME: 5 minutes • **COOK TIME:** 45 minutes

If you're like me and love savory crunchy snacks, then this recipe is perfect for you. These roasted chickpeas are a great alternative to salty processed potato chips. They are easily customizable to your specific cravings: Try lemon pepper, garlic seasoning, or Cajun seasoning.

2 (15-ounce) cans no-salt-added chickpeas, drained, rinsed, and patted dry

Avocado or olive oil cooking spray

2 tablespoons Barbecue Rub Seasoning Blend (page 137) or store-bought

1. Preheat the oven to 350°F. Line a baking sheet with parchment paper.

2. Pour the chickpeas onto the prepared baking sheet and spray lightly with cooking spray. Sprinkle the seasoning on the chickpeas. Toss gently to coat.

3. Bake for about 45 minutes, until brown and crispy. You want to stir the pan every 15 to 20 minutes to prevent any burning.

4. Store leftovers in bowl with a paper towel draped over them or in glass container with the lid slightly ajar for 1 to 2 days.

PER SERVING (½ CUP): Calories: 202; Protein: 10.1g; Carbohydrates: 33g; Fiber: 9g; Total Fat 4g; Saturated Fat: 0g; Sodium: 16mg; Cholesterol: 0mg; Potassium: 188mg; Phosphorus: 123mg

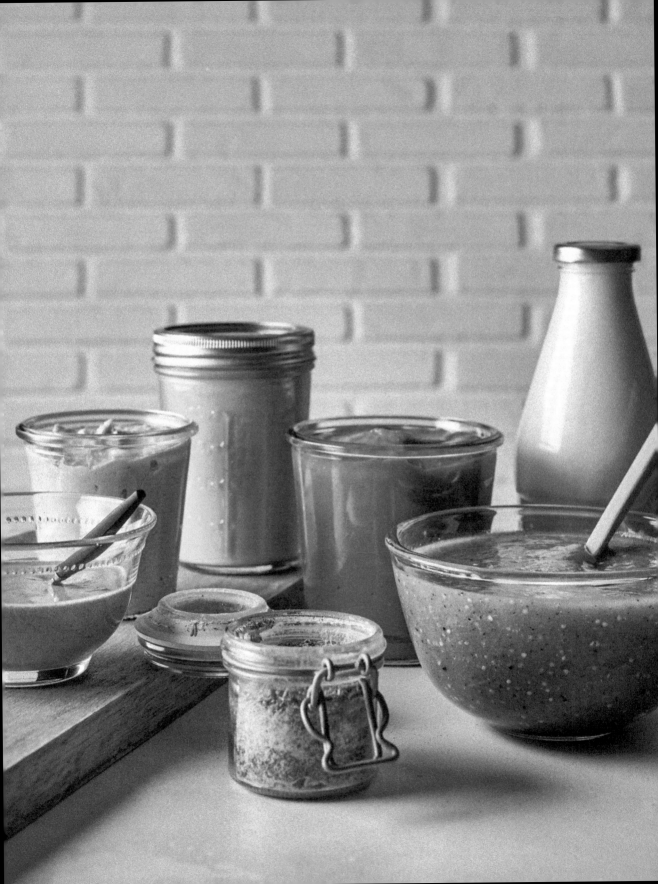

8

Staples and Seasonings

Taco Seasoning

DIABETES-FRIENDLY • HEART-HEALTHY • LOW-PROTEIN • ONE POT

MAKES 4 TABLESPOONS • PREP TIME: 5 minutes

Premade Mexican-blend taco seasonings tend to have extra salt and other additives that you don't want when eating a kidney-friendly diet. Making your own at home is super easy and cost effective. Customize it by adjusting the levels of different spices depending on your taste preferences. This seasoning mix is great on many dishes such as tacos, on meats, or even salads.

1 tablespoon ground cumin

2 teaspoons paprika

2 teaspoons garlic powder

2 teaspoons freshly ground black pepper

1 teaspoon dried oregano

1 teaspoon red pepper flakes

½ teaspoon ground cinnamon

½ teaspoon onion powder

1. In a sealable container, combine the cumin, paprika, garlic powder, black pepper, oregano, red pepper flakes, cinnamon, and onion powder and mix well.

2. This seasoning can be stored in an airtight container at room temperature for up to 1 year. Label and date before storing.

PER SERVING (1 TABLESPOON): Calories: 20; Protein: 0.9g; Carbohydrates: 4g; Fiber 1g; Total Fat: 1g; Saturated Fat: 0g; Sodium: 5mg; Cholesterol: 0mg; Potassium: 95mg; Phosphorus: 21mg

Curry Garlic Seasoning

DIABETES-FRIENDLY • HEART-HEALTHY • LOW-PROTEIN
ONE POT • 5 INGREDIENTS OR FEWER

MAKES 10 TABLESPOONS • **PREP TIME:** 5 minutes

I love eating curry dishes and there are so many different varieties from different countries. Though it's convenient to use prepackaged curry flavorings, they are often full of sodium and other additives. This seasoning blend is great in stews, Mediterranean dishes, wraps, sandwiches, roasted vegetables, and more! I like to add a spicy kick to it by using red pepper flakes as well.

4 tablespoons dried onion flakes

3 tablespoons garlic powder

1½ tablespoons curry powder

½ tablespoon freshly ground black pepper

⅛ teaspoon ground cayenne pepper

1. In a sealable container, combine the onion flakes, garlic powder, curry powder, black pepper, and cayenne and mix well.

2. This seasoning can be stored at room temperature for up to 1 year. Label and date before storing.

PER SERVING (1 TABLESPOON): Calories: 21; Protein: 0.8g; Carbohydrates: 5g; Fiber 1g; Total Fat: 0g; Saturated Fat: 0g; Sodium: 3mg; Cholesterol: 0mg; Potassium: 83mg; Phosphorus: 22mg

Italian Seasoning Blend

DIABETES-FRIENDLY • HEART-HEALTHY • LOW-PROTEIN • ONE POT

MAKES 8 TABLESPOONS • **PREP TIME:** 5 minutes

Italian seasoning blend is super easy to make and you likely already have all the ingredients in your pantry. This type of seasoning blend is often used to flavor many Italian dishes such as pizza, pasta, soups, vegetables, and even meat dishes. I love adding the optional red pepper flakes to give it an extra kick and add some pizzazz.

2 tablespoons dried basil

2 tablespoons dried oregano

2 tablespoons dried parsley

1 tablespoon dried rosemary

1 tablespoon dried thyme

1 tablespoon red pepper flakes (optional)

2 teaspoons garlic powder

1. In a sealable container, combine the basil, oregano, parsley, rosemary, thyme, red pepper flakes (if using), and garlic powder and mix well.

2. This seasoning can be stored at room temperature for up to 1 year. Label and date before storing.

PER SERVING (1 TABLESPOON): Calories: 9; Protein: 0.5g; Carbohydrates: 2g; Fiber 1g; Total Fat: 0g; Saturated Fat: 0g; Sodium: 3mg; Cholesterol: 0mg; Potassium: 49mg; Phosphorus: 8mg

Barbecue Rub Seasoning Blend

DIABETES-FRIENDLY • HEART-HEALTHY • LOW-PROTEIN • ONE POT

MAKES 4 TABLESPOONS • PREP TIME: 5 minutes

Barbecue always reminds me of holidays and fun parties with family and friends. I love that this rub is so easy to make and can be used in so many different recipes. Commercially made barbecue rubs and sauces are often jam-packed with extra sodium and sugars. This easy homemade recipe is low in sodium and loaded with flavor. I use it as a rub on meats, sprinkled over vegetables, and in the Barbecue Roasted Chickpeas (page 130).

1 tablespoon
brown sugar

1 teaspoon
smoked paprika

1 teaspoon chili powder

1 teaspoon
garlic powder

1 teaspoon
onion powder

1 teaspoon
ground cumin

¼ teaspoon dry mustard

⅛ teaspoon allspice

⅛ teaspoon red pepper
flakes (optional)

1. In an airtight container, combine the brown sugar, paprika, chili powder, garlic powder, onion powder, cumin, mustard, allspice, and red pepper flakes (if using) and mix well.

2. This seasoning can be stored at room temperature for up to 1 year. Label and date before storing.

PER SERVING (1 TABLESPOON): Calories: 16; Protein: 0.4g; Carbohydrates: 4g; Fiber 0g; Total Fat: 0g; Saturated Fat: 0g; Sodium: 18mg; Cholesterol: 0mg; Potassium: 29mg; Phosphorus: 9mg

Roasted Tomatillo Salsa

DIABETES-FRIENDLY • HEART-HEALTHY • LOW-PROTEIN

MAKES 2 CUPS • **PREP TIME:** 5 minutes • **COOK TIME:** 15 minutes

Salsas tend to get a bad reputation in the kidney realm due to their potassium content. Hopefully, you've learned by now that potassium may not need to be restricted when you have CKD. This homemade salsa is low in sodium and packed with tons of flavor. I love to use this on almost everything—it's perfect with crackers, corn chips, over tacos, on salads, and more.

16 tomatillos, halved

3 jalapeños, stemmed

10 garlic cloves, peeled

2 tablespoons avo-
cado oil, plus more for
drizzling

1 bunch fresh cilantro

¼ cup freshly squeezed
lime juice

¼ cup water

1. Preheat the broiler to high and line a baking sheet with parchment paper.

2. Spread the tomatillos, jalapeños, and garlic on the baking sheet. Drizzle with oil and toss gently to coat.

3. Broil for 10 to 15 minutes, until the tomatillos are browned. Transfer the ingredients, along with the cilantro, lime juice, water, and avocado oil to a food processor or blender and puree until smooth.

4. Store leftovers in an airtight container in the refrigerator for up to 7 days. Cool completely, label, and date before storing.

PER SERVING (¼ CUP): Calories: 22; Protein: 0.7g;
Carbohydrates: 4g; Fiber 1g; Total Fat: 1g; Saturated Fat: 0g;
Sodium: 1mg; Cholesterol: 0mg; Potassium: 182mg; Phosphorus: 27mg

Low-Sodium Dijon Mustard

DIABETES-FRIENDLY • HEART-HEALTHY • LOW-PROTEIN

MAKES 12 TEASPOONS • **PREP TIME:** 5 minutes

Mustard is one of the oldest condiments, which was first used by the Romans in the 10th century—and it's one of my favorite condiments. Mustard has a tangy and pungent taste and I love to use it on sandwiches, burgers, as a dip for veggies, and mixed into dressings and sauces. You will find many of the recipes in this book use this mustard for flavoring. When you buy prepacked mustard, it is usually high in sodium and also has added sugars, both of which you want to limit when following a healthy diet.

1 cup dry white wine

½ cup white vinegar

¼ cup chopped onion

½ tablespoon sugar

2 garlic cloves, minced

1 teaspoon allspice

1 bay leaf

½ teaspoon dried tarragon

¼ teaspoon ground cayenne pepper

¼ cup cold water

½ cup dry mustard

1. In a medium saucepan, combine the wine, vinegar, onion, sugar, garlic, allspice, bay leaf, tarragon, and cayenne over medium-high heat.

2. Boil the mixture until reduced by half, about 20 minutes.

3. Meanwhile, in a large bowl, combine the water and the mustard and let sit for 10 minutes. Strain the vinegar mixture into the mustard mixture and stir.

4. Return the mix to the saucepan and cook over medium-low heat for an additional 10 minutes, stirring frequently.

5. This mustard can be stored in the refrigerator for up to 3 months. Cool completely, label, and date before storing.

PER SERVING (1 TEASPOON): Calories: 39; Protein: 1.2g; Carbohydrates: 3g; Fiber 1g; Total Fat: 2g; Saturated Fat: 0g; Sodium: 6mg; Cholesterol: 0mg; Potassium: 51mg; Phosphorus: 39mg

Mango Teriyaki Sauce

DIABETES-FRIENDLY • HEART-HEALTHY • LOW-PROTEIN

MAKES 1¼ CUPS • PREP TIME: 5 minutes • **COOK TIME:** 30 minutes

Growing up, I loved eating chicken or salmon with teriyaki sauce and I often drenched my food in the sauce. Though they sell teriyaki sauce premade in stores, it is often filled with excess amounts of sugar and sodium. This recipe is a more nutritious version as it uses fruits (dates and mango) to create that sweet flavor. If you don't have mango, you can also use pineapple (fresh, canned, or frozen) to make this delicious sauce.

3 Medjool dates, pitted

2 cups water

½ cup chopped mango

1 tablespoon low-sodium soy sauce

1 tablespoon sesame oil

1 teaspoon rice wine vinegar

¼ teaspoon ground ginger

¼ teaspoon garlic powder

1. In a small bowl, cover the dates with the water and let sit for 15 minutes. Reserve 1 cup of the liquid and drain the dates.

2. In a blender or food processor, combine the dates and reserved water, mango, soy sauce, sesame oil, vinegar, ginger, and garlic powder and puree until smooth.

3. Pour the sauce into a saucepan and bring to a boil over medium heat. Once boiling, remove from the heat and let simmer, stirring occasionally. The sauce should thicken up in 10 to 15 minutes.

4. Store leftovers in an airtight container in the refrigerator for up to 7 days.

PER SERVING (1 TABLESPOON): Calories: 20; Protein: 0.2g; Carbohydrates: 4g; Fiber 0g; Total Fat: 1g; Saturated Fat: 0g; Sodium: 24mg; Cholesterol: 0mg; Potassium: 37mg; Phosphorus: 4mg

Peanut Apple Sauce

MAKES 8 TABLESPOONS • PREP TIME: 5 minutes

Peanut sauces are used in many different Asian cuisines. I love the nutty and sweet flavor of those dishes. This recipe is great because it uses natural ingredients to create the same flavors. Use this sauce on noodle or rice dishes and as a dipping sauce or marinade for proteins and vegetables. You can also use chunky peanut butter to add a crunchy texture.

¼ cup creamy unsalted peanut butter

3 to 4 tablespoons warm water

2 tablespoons unsweetened applesauce

1 tablespoon rice vinegar

¼ teaspoon ground ginger

1. In a small bowl or jar, mix the peanut butter, warm water, applesauce, vinegar, and ginger until well combined. Store in an airtight container.

2. Store leftovers in the refrigerator in an airtight container for up to 7 days.

PER SERVING (1 TABLESPOON): Calories: 50; Protein: 0.4g; Carbohydrates: 2g; Fiber 1g; Total Fat: 4g; Saturated Fat: 1g; Sodium: 2mg; Cholesterol: 0mg; Potassium: 4mg; Phosphorus: 0mg

Enchilada Sauce

DIABETES-FRIENDLY • HEART-HEALTHY • LOW-PROTEIN

MAKES 3 CUPS • PREP TIME: 5 minutes • **COOK TIME:** 20 minutes

This sauce is packed with flavor and free from unnecessary ingredients. Premade enchilada sauce often has way too much salt and other processed ingredients or additives. I love the rich umami flavor of this sauce and am amazed that I can create it with many pantry staples.

2 tablespoons all-purpose flour

8 ounces no-salt-added tomato sauce

2 tablespoons no-salt-added tomato paste

2 tablespoons olive or avocado oil

1 tablespoon chili powder

1 teaspoon ground cumin

1 teaspoon garlic powder

½ teaspoon dried oregano

¼ teaspoon ground cinnamon

2 cups no-salt-added vegetable broth

1. In a medium saucepan, heat the flour over medium-high heat and whisk for a minute to heat it up. Stir in the tomato sauce, tomato paste, oil, chili powder, cumin, garlic powder, oregano, and cinnamon.

2. Add the broth in ½-cup increments to the mixture, stirring constantly. Reduce the heat and let simmer for 10 to 15 minutes until thickened.

3. Store leftovers in an airtight container in the refrigerator for up to 7 days.

PER SERVING (½ CUP): Calories: 80; Protein: 2.2g; Carbohydrates: 8g; Fiber 2g; Total Fat: 5g; Saturated Fat: 1g; Sodium: 66mg; Cholesterol: 2mg; Potassium: 268mg; Phosphorus: 22mg

Unsweetened Almond Milk

DIABETES-FRIENDLY • HEART-HEALTHY • 5 INGREDIENTS OR FEWER

MAKES 3 CUPS • PREP TIME: 10 minutes, plus 8 to 12 hours to soak

Commercially prepared almond milk usually contains excess salt and other additives, including potassium or phosphate. Homemade nut milk is a better option with less additives and it is more affordable, too! You can mix in different flavorings based on your preferences. I like to mix it up by using vanilla, cinnamon, maple syrup, or cacao powder. You can use other types of nuts to vary the flavor of the nut milk. Try cashews, walnuts, or hazelnuts.

1 cup raw almonds

3 cups filtered water, plus more for soaking

1. Pour the almonds in a quart jar and add enough water to cover the almonds. Set in the refrigerator to soak for 6 to 8 hours or overnight.

2. Drain the almonds and transfer to a blender. Pour in the filtered water and blend on high until the almonds are finely ground and the liquid is white.

3. Put a cheesecloth over a strainer set on a large bowl. Working in batches, pour the almond mixture into the cheesecloth, squeezing the cheesecloth to extract all the liquid. Discard the almond pulp.

4. Add any flavorings, if desired. Store in an airtight container in the refrigerator for up to 3 days.

PER SERVING (1 CUP): Calories: 40; Protein: 1g; Carbohydrates: 2g; Fiber 0 g; Total Fat: 3g; Saturated Fat: 0g; Sodium: 6mg; Cholesterol: 0mg; Potassium: 180mg; Phosphorus: 40mg

Salt-Free Pizza Dough

DIABETES-FRIENDLY • HEART-HEALTHY • LOW-PROTEIN
ONE POT • 5-INGREDIENTS OR FEWER

MAKES 12 SLICES • PREP TIME: 45 minutes • **COOK TIME:** 25 minutes

Pizza dough is surprisingly easy to make. Homemade pizza dough tastes much better than store-bought, and my kids and I have so much fun creating our own pizzas. You can even add some seasonings, like Italian Seasoning Blend (page 136), to add more flavor.

1 cup warm water (temperature should be between 105°F and 110°F)

1 tablespoon sugar

1¼ teaspoons active dry yeast

2 tablespoons olive or avocado oil, divided

2½ cups all-purpose flour, divided, plus more for dusting

1. In a large mixing bowl, combine the warm water, sugar, and yeast. Stir to combine.

2. When it starts to bubble and froth, after 5 to 10 minutes, add 1 tablespoon of oil and stir gently to combine. Add 2 cups of flour and gently stir to form a soft dough.

3. Transfer the dough onto a floured surface and knead until it is smooth and no longer sticky. You may need to add more flour. Try ½ tablespoon at a time, up to ½ cup, until you achieve the desired consistency.

4. Grease the bowl with the remaining 1 tablespoon of oil and turn the dough to grease all sides. Cover the dough and let sit in a warm area for 30 minutes.

5. Transfer the dough back onto a floured surface and form it into whatever shape you like. Roll it out until it is about ½ inch thick. If you'd like to have a crust, fold over the edges.

6. Prebake the crust in the oven for about 5 minutes before adding your toppings. Remove from the heat, add your desired toppings, and return to the oven on the lower rack to cook for about 20 minutes, until golden and cooked through.

PER SERVING (1 SLICE): Calories: 91; Protein: 2.3g; Carbohydrates: 17g; Fiber 1g; Total Fat: 1g; Saturated Fat: 0g; Sodium: 2mg; Cholesterol: 0mg; Potassium: 28 mg; Phosphorus: 26 mg

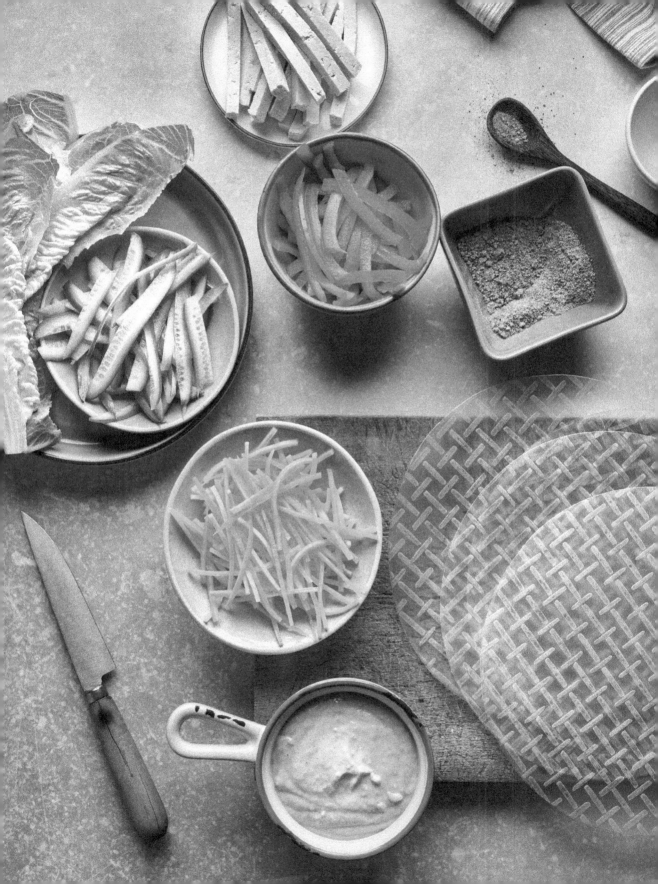

Measurement Conversions

Volume Equivalents (Liquid)

US STANDARD	US STANDARD (OUNCES)	METRIC (APPROXIMATE)
2 tablespoons	1 fl. oz.	30 mL
¼ cup	2 fl. oz.	60 mL
½ cup	4 fl. oz.	120 mL
1 cup	8 fl. oz.	240 mL
1½ cups	12 fl. oz.	355 mL
2 cups or 1 pint	16 fl. oz.	475 mL
4 cups or 1 quart	32 fl. oz.	1 L
1 gallon	128 fl. oz.	4 L

Oven Temperatures

FAHRENHEIT (F)	CELSIUS (C) (APPROXIMATE)
250°F	120°C
300°F	150°C
325°F	165°C
350°F	180°C
375°F	190°C
400°F	200°C
425°F	220°C
450°F	230°C

Volume Equivalents (Dry)

US STANDARD	METRIC (APPROXIMATE)
⅛ teaspoon	0.5 mL
¼ teaspoon	1 mL
½ teaspoon	2 mL
¾ teaspoon	4 mL
1 teaspoon	5 mL
1 tablespoon	15 mL
¼ cup	59 mL
⅓ cup	79 mL
½ cup	118 mL
⅔ cup	156 mL
¾ cup	177 mL
1 cup	235 mL
2 cups or 1 pint	475 mL
3 cups	700 mL
4 cups or 1 quart	1 L

Weight Equivalents

US STANDARD	METRIC (APPROXIMATE)
½ ounce	15 g
1 ounce	30 g
2 ounces	60 g
4 ounces	115 g
8 ounces	225 g
12 ounces	340 g
16 ounces or 1 pound	455 g

Resources

Centers for Disease Control and Prevention, Chronic Kidney Disease Initiative

CDC.gov/kidneydisease

The CDC's website includes information on promoting kidney health, preventing and controlling risk factors for CKD, and raising awareness on diagnosis and treatments.

DaVita Kidney Care

DaVita.com

Worldwide dialysis company with information on kidney disease, dialysis, and nutrition.

Edith Yang, RD, CSR, CLT, Healthy Mission Dietitian, Inc.

HealthyMissionDietitian.com

One-on-one nutrition counseling with a board-certified renal registered dietitian.

Find a CKD Dietitian

Sites.google.com/view/ckdrd/home

Resource to find a dietitian specializing in kidney disease near you.

Find a Registered Dietitian Nutritionist

EatRight.org/find-an-expert

Resource to find a registered dietitian near you.

Flavis

Flavis.com/en

Food products for those with chronic kidney disease.

Fresenius Kidney Care

FreseniusKidneyCare.com

Worldwide dialysis company with information on kidney disease, dialysis, and nutrition.

Kidney Disease Improving Global Outcomes (KDIGO)

KDIGO.org

KDIGO is a global nonprofit organization that provides evidence-based guidelines for practice to clinicians and patients with kidney disease.

National Institute of Diabetes and Digestive and Kidney Diseases

NIDDK.nih.gov

Information and education on diabetes and kidney disease from the National Institute of Health.

National Kidney Foundation

Kidney.org

A national resource for patients to learn more about kidney disease and a place where they can get support and connect with others.

Satellite Healthcare

SatelliteHealth.com

National dialysis company with information on kidney disease and dialysis.

USDA Food Database

FDC.nal.usda.gov

Resource on the nutritional content information on foods.

US Renal Care

USRenalCare.com

National dialysis company with information on kidney disease, dialysis, and nutrition.

US Food and Drug Administration, Food Labeling and Nutrition

FDA.gov/food/food-labeling-nutrition

Information on the new food labels and how to read them.

2015–2020 Dietary Guidelines for Americans

DietaryGuidelines.gov/current-dietary-guidelines/2015-2020-dietary-guidelines

Diet and lifestyle recommendations for Americans.

References

Bethke, P. C., and S. H. Jansky. "The Effects of Boiling and Leaching on the Content of Potassium and Other Minerals in Potatoes." *Journal of Food Science* 73, no. 5 (June/July 2008): H80–H85. doi.org/10.1111/j.1750-3841.2008.00782.x.

Bouhairie, Victoria E., and Janet B. McGill. "Diabetic Kidney Disease." *Missouri Medicine* 113, no. 5 (September–October 2016): 390–394. ncbi.nlm.nih.gov/pmc /articles/PMC6139827.

Byham-Gray, Laura, Jean Stover, and Karen Wiesen, eds. *A Clinical Guide to Nutrition Care in Kidney Disease*. 2nd ed. Chicago, IL: Academy of Nutrition and Dietetics, 2013.

Centers for Disease Control and Prevention. "Chronic Kidney Disease in the United States, 2019." Accessed February 24, 2021. CDC.gov/kidneydisease/publications -resources/2019-national-facts.html.

Dietary Guidelines for Americans. "Current Dietary Guidelines." Accessed February 2, 2021. dietaryguidelines.gov/current-dietary-guidelines/2015-2020 -dietary-guidelines.

Forouhi, Nita G., Ronald M. Krauss, Gary Taubes, and Walter Willett. "Dietary Fat and Cardiometabolic Health: Evidence, Controversies, and Consensus for Guidance." *BMJ* 2018, no. 361 (June 13, 2018): k2139. doi.org/10.1136/bmj.k2139.

Fu, Haiyan, Silvia Liu, Sheldon I. Bastacky, Xiaojie Wang, Xiao-Jun Tian, and Dong Zhou. "Diabetic Kidney Diseases Revisited: A New Perspective for a New Era." *Molecular Metabolism* 30 (December 2019): 250–263. doi.org/10.1016 /j.molmet.2019.10.005.

Ikizler, T. Alp, Jerrilynn D. Burrowes, Laura D. Byham-Gray, Katrina L. Campbell, Juan-Jesus Carrero, Winnie Chan, and Denis Fouque, et al. "Clinical Practice Guideline for Nutrition in Chronic Kidney Disease: 2019 Update." *National Kidney Foundation*. Published October 2019. kidney.org/sites/default/files /Nutrition_GL%2BSubmission_101719_Public_Review_Copy.pdf.

Katz, David L., Kim Doughty, and Ather Ali. "Cocoa and Chocolate in Human Health and Disease." *Antioxidants & Redox Signaling* 15, no. 10 (November 15, 2011): 2779–2811. doi.org/10.1089/ars.2010.3697.

Ko, Gang Jee, Yoshitsugu Obi, Amanda R. Tortorici, and Kamyar Kalantar-Zadeh. "Dietary Protein Intake and Chronic Kidney Disease." *Current Opinion in Clinical Nutrition and Metabolic Care* 20, no. 1 (January 2017), 77–85. doi.org/10.1097/MCO.0000000000000342.

Kramer, Holly. "Diet and Chronic Kidney Disease." *Advances in Nutrition* 10, supplement no. 4 (November 2019): S367–S379. doi.org/10.1093/advances/nmz011.

Orth, Stephan R., and Stein I. Hallan. "Smoking: A Risk Factor for Progression of Chronic Kidney Disease and for Cardiovascular Morbidity and Mortality in Renal Patients—Absence of Evidence or Evidence of Absence?" *Clinical Journal of the American Society of Nephrology* 3, no. 1 (January 2008): 226–236. doi.org/10.2215/CJN.03740907.

Poole, Robin, Oliver J. Kennedy, Paul Roderick, Jonathan A. Fallowfield, Peter C. Hayes, and Julie Parkes. "Coffee Consumption and Health: Umbrella Review of Meta-Analyses of Multiple Health Outcomes." *BMJ* 2017, no. 359 (November 22, 2017). bmj.com/content/359/bmj.j5024.

Ritz, E., K. Hahn, M. Ketteler, M. K. Kuhlmann, and J. Mann. "Phosphate Additives in Food: A Health Risk." *Deutsches Ärzteblatt International* 109, no. 4 (2012): 49–55. doi.org/10.3238/arztebl.2012.0049.

US Department of Agriculture. "FoodData Central." (n.d.). fdc.nal.usda.gov.

Viana, João L., George C. Kosmadakis, Emma L. Watson, Alan Bevington, John Feehally, Nicolette C. Bishop, and Alice C. Smith. "Evidence for Anti-Inflammatory Effects of Exercise in CKD." *Journal of the American Society of Nephrology* 25, no. 9 (September 2014): 2121–2130. doi.org/10.1681/ASN.2013070702.

Wright, Julie A., and Kerri L. Cavanaugh. "Dietary Sodium in Chronic Kidney Disease: A Comprehensive Approach." *Seminars in Dialysis* 23, no. 4 (July/August 2010): 415–21. doi.org/10.1111/j.1525-139X.2010.00752.x.

Index

H

Acknowledgments

I'd like to thank my husband for being my biggest fan and supporting me through this endeavor, and for being my primary taste tester. A big thank-you to my daughters, Penelope and Charlotte. Penny: You are so sweet, thoughtful, strong, brave, and an amazing big sister; thank you for being so patient. Charlotte: You timed things better than I ever could have imagined; thank you for being such a sweetheart and so easygoing.

Thank you to my parents for always supporting me and allowing me to pursue my life goals and desires. I'd also like to thank my parents as well as my in-laws for helping me entertain my children as I secretly write a cookbook.

Thank you to my colleagues and friends Nancy, Jessica, and Connie for their constant love, encouragement, and support.

Thank you to my editor, Rachelle, and the team at Callisto Media for giving me the opportunity to write a cookbook and supporting me throughout the entire process.

Finally, a big thank-you to all my clients for being my inspiration for this cookbook.

About the Author

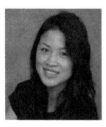

EDITH YANG, RD, CSR, CLT, is a registered dietitian board-certified in renal nutrition, a certified LEAP therapist, and the owner of Healthy Mission Dietitian, Inc. Edith has experience working with a variety of patients and is passionate about all things related to food. Her goal is to teach and empower people to properly fuel and nourish their bodies to live happy, healthy lives and prevent many chronic illnesses. Edith is based in Los Angeles, California, where she lives with her husband and two daughters. She enjoys spending time with her family, exploring Los Angeles and eating her way through the city. For more information on Edith, her practice, and working with her, visit her at HealthyMissionDietitian.com.

CPSIA information can be obtained
at www.ICGtesting.com
Printed in the USA
JSHW022303050921
18424JS00001B/1